DETOX
NATURALLY

Rajgopal Nidamboor

Emerald Publishing
www.emeraldpublishing.co.uk

Emerald Guides
Brighton BN2 4EG

First published 2010
© Rajgopal Nidamboor

ISBN 9781847161697
Printed by GN Digital Printing Essex
Cover design by Bookworks Islington London
Author's photograph by Yashwant Rao

While every effort has been made to ensure that the information contained within this book is correct at the time of going to press, the author and publisher can take no responsibility for the errors, or omissions, contained therein.

Disclaimer: The information presented in this work is in no way intended as medical advice and/or as a substitute for medical treatment. Nothing in this work is intended to self-diagnose, or self-treat, any illness/disease/health condition. The publisher, author, and retailer of this work accept no responsibility for personal injury, or mechanical damage, which may result from using this work. Should the reader have any questions, or queries, concerning the appropriateness of any therapy, procedure, method, or preparation mentioned, the publisher and the author strongly recommend seeking the counsel/advice of a professional physician/therapist/healthcare adviser/provider.

Contents

Contents

Contents

Contents

INTRODUCTION

"I believe that you can, by taking some simple and inexpensive measures, extend your life and your years of well-being. My most important recommendation is that you take vitamins every day in optimum amounts, to supplement the vitamins you receive in your food…"

"… Chelation therapy is far safer and much less expensive than surgical treatment of atherosclerosis. Chelation therapy might eliminate the need for bypass surgery and is equally valid when used as a preventative treatment."

— Linus Pauling, PhD, the only two-time Nobel laureate

Ever thought of a non-surgical procedure that was safe, economical, and easy-to-use, to circumvent the need for bypass, angioplasty, or stents?

If you haven't, there's no need to search the horizons — because, there is!

For good measure, it has proven benefits — based on actual patient results and studies conducted during the past five decades. Its name: chelation therapy.

Chelation therapy is a simple form of medical treatment that not only reverses and slows down the progression of atherosclerosis, but also stalls the development of other age-related and degenerative diseases. There is also an additional benefit. The therapy improves symptoms associated with many other diseases affecting the body, though why this happens is not yet fully understood — but, the best part, which is also the most important and verifiable aspect of the chelation treatment plan, is it happens.

A non-invasive form of treatment, chelation [pronounced, *key-lay-shun*] therapy is resourcefully used today in the treatment of atherosclerosis and other chronic degenerative diseases involving the circulatory system, besides a host of functional and pathological disorders, including the removal of toxic effects of metals.

Atherosclerosis — hardening of the arteries — is a progressive disease. It is characterised by irregularly distributed lipid [cholesterol] deposits in large and medium-sized arteries. Lipid deposits are associated with fibrosis [formation of fibrous tissue as a reparative or reactive process, as opposed to the formation of fibrous tissue as a normal constituent of an organ or tissue], and calcification [deposition of lime, or insoluble calcium salts]. Over a period of time, the condition can lead to heart attacks.

Studies also suggest that following the use of the chelation procedure blood flow increases not only in the blocked coronary arteries to the heart, but also the brain, the legs, and elsewhere in the body. This explains why heart attacks, strokes, leg pain and gangrene [disease due to reduced blood supply, or obstruction], can be avoided through chelation therapy.

Likewise, the need for bypass surgery, and angioplasty, can also be avoided with this effective therapy, before things go too far.
This is not all. Experts suggest that chelation therapy acts as a preventative aid against cancer.

One of the most important benefits of chelation therapy — which has also been scientifically demonstrated — is its ground-breaking effects on the free radical foundation of disease and its annihilation.

Free radicals are highly unstable chemicals that attack, infiltrate, and injure vital cell structures.

Many scientific studies provide adequate clinical evidence of this benefit, among a host of other advantages, by way of chelation therapy. Experts also suggest that since chelation therapy is a non-invasive technique, it is much safer and less expensive than conventional or advanced surgery, including bypass and angioplasty.

Statistics indicates that over 700,000 individuals have undergone chelation therapy since its inception over fifty years ago, without a single loss of life due to complications. What's more, the American College of Advancement of Medicine [ACAM] estimates that approximately 600,000 patients have received over 10,000,000 chelation treatments — without a single fatality being attributed to the use of EDTA [ethylene-diamine-tetra-acetic acid], the premier chelating agent in use.

Is this not a stunning safety record for a medical procedure — something that no surgical procedure, or even the "wonder drug" aspirin can match?

****

Chapter 1

WHAT IS CHELATION?

Chelation traces its origins from the Greek word, *chele*. Its English corollary is "claw" — something you'd refer to a scorpion's line of attack or defence.

The concept *per se* is based on the study that when a certain amino acid complex called EDTA [ethylene-diamine-tetra-acetic acid] comes in contact with certain positively charged metals and other substances, such as lead, iron, copper, calcium, magnesium, zinc, plutonium and manganese, it clasps them and eliminates them. You got it. Hence, the word — *chele* or chelation — a process of eradicating unwanted ionic material from the body by the infusion of EDTA, an organic compound, which has suitable chelating properties.

In other words, EDTA grabs metallic cations such as calcium from the body. In the process, it forms a stable compound, which is subsequently excreted from the system. It must also be mentioned that the stability of this binding mechanism is crucial in chelation therapy, and also its successful application. If the bond is fragile, other chemicals can sever the "connection" and form their own compounds.

EDTA is a synthetic amino acid. It was first used for the treatment of heavy metal poisoning in the 1940s, It is widely recognised to be just as useful in a variety of conditions, including emergency treatment of hypercalcaemia [abnormally high concentration of calcium compounds in the circulating blood], and the control of ventricular arrhythmias [rhythmic disturbance of the heart] associated with digitalis [a drug used in heart affections] toxicity.

In the 1960s, EDTA was also found to be quite effective in the treatment of occlusive vascular disorders caused by the hardening of arteries, or atherosclerosis, according to studies conducted at the National Academy of Sciences, US.

Simple premise, profound effect

You could think of the chelation process as something we often do to clear our drainage system. When a drain is clogged, we add a chemical. The substance dissolves the blockage. Soon after, the resulting compound is also removed from the drain through the plumbing system. Chelation process works, more or less, in the same manner in our body.

Our digestive process is an excellent example of the chelation process. Just think of the biological blueprint of digestion and assimilation of food. This is similar to the chelation process of amino acids, or proteins, and minerals — to which blood cells fasten to obtain iron. Iron is fundamental for the transportation of nutrients within the body.

To use a simile. Green vegetables contain iron. When we consume them, our digestive process releases the iron to which it is bound. Iron needs to be chelated, or combined, with amino acids and carried through the intestinal mucous membranes into the bloodstream.

Another great example is tea, especially green tea [distilled in water, without milk and sugar]. When we drink the brew that cheers, with a meal, as is the custom in China, the tannin content in tea will chelate with iron to form iron tannate — a non-soluble compound — before it gets engaged to be flushed out of the body.

The whole process is, of course, dependent on our nutritional intake, especially foods rich in vitamin C — or, supplements — and, iron. Vitamin C chelates with iron; it boosts and quickens the absorption of iron. Once iron enters the bloodstream, it is freed from the proteins to which it was chelated during the course of its journey.

To mirror another example. As you may well know, haemoglobin is a "chelate" of iron. Haemoglobin transports oxygen from the lungs to the tissues. When haemoglobin is exposed to certain chemicals, its normal respiratory function is blocked.

Yet another useful example is the enzyme catalase, a natural chelating agent, which is used by our body to untangle the free radical activity of hydrogen peroxide, an unstable compound.

Other uses

Apart from its usefulness in the treatment of atherosclerosis and other chronic degenerative diseases involving the circulatory system, as outlined earlier, chelation therapy offers many other benefits.

Experts suggest that chelation can quite easily remove metallic catalysts that cause excessive free radical proliferation. This, in turn, reduces the oxidation of lipids [cholesterol], or fats, DNA, enzyme systems and lipoproteins, or complexes or compounds containing lipids and proteins. There you are — chelation therapy not only "freezes" the bad effects but also spurs the body's healing process to reverse any damage caused by free radicals.

Chelation therapy can help remove calcium and copper anions from the blood stream. Remember, these anions can make the plaque lining the artery walls "jammed" and weak. Chelation therapy can get them extricated.

Just think of the benefits — even if chelation can purge just a small layer of plaque formation, as some critics imply, it can improve the blood flow to the arteries significantly. This action, by itself, can avert arterial spasm and minimise and/or even prevent anginal pain. What's more, chelation can also make the artery wall pliant. In so doing, it can provide the healing touch to the cells that line the arteries.

Angina is a severe constricting pain in the chest, often radiating from the precordium [the epigastrium and anterior surface of the lower part of the thorax] to the left shoulder and down the arm, due to ischaemia [narrowing] of the heart muscle, usually caused by coronary disease. As a matter of fact, patients have reported that they can walk without anginal pain after chelation therapy — something they could just not think of doing earlier.

"Oatvantage"

The current popular trend for oat-based foods as a means of reducing cholesterol levels is but one form of chelation therapy, which we take for granted. In fact, the different forms of fibre found in food, such as soluble pectin in apples and other fruits, guar in beans as well as fibre found in grains, all produce multiple chelating effects as they pass through the system. They act largely in the bowel where they speed up transit time and, in the process, prevent cholesterol reabsorption from the bile. This is said to clear the waste material from the system more rapidly. Fats in the bloodstream are also, likewise, reduced by soluble fibre in the diet. This further helps to decrease the potential for free radical activity.

An ideal form of diet, or what is called as balanced diet, can easily produce natural chelation effects when followed conscientiously. In addition, many basic nutrients such as vitamins C and E are natural chelators; in ample supply, they dampen down free radical activity and also chelate toxic substances in the bloodstream.

Several health formulae have been developed for oral chelation using variable combinations of substances. Some are extremely complex and others simple enough to piece together in formulations. All one needs to possess is a little patience and sound advice from a chelation specialist to derive maximum benefits from this simple, non-invasive and effective therapy.

Historical background

When Alfred Werner, a pioneering biochemist, developed the theory of co-ordination compounds, in 1893, which is now called chelates, there was not much to co-ordination compounds than what meets treatment plans today. That Werner received the Nobel Prize for reclassifying inorganic chemical compounds, was more than a milestone — it's an outcome that prompted him to formulate an accounting system for the process by which metals are attached to organic molecules. This was, indeed, the foundation of chelation therapy.

Werner's monumental discovery was first used in the industrial sector. A few years down the line, many new materials, such as paint, were launched. Gradually, it was found that the elimination of heavy metal contamination, during the manufacturing process, was mandatory, and for good reasons. Citric acid was soon found to be helpful in achieving this objective.

It was at this point of time that the growing aspirations of a handful of scientists in Germany to find something new, led to the development of a new chelating material that was not dependent on citric acid, or its import. The synthetic substance the intrepid Germans invented was none other than the famed EDTA. EDTA was created for Germany's own use, to "beat" citric acid imports, but thanks to surplus production, the product gained such a reputation that German exports spiralled — they began selling it in bulk for industrial use worldwide.

Although medical applications were not, at this point of time, considered for EDTA, World War II spawned a new line of thought. As army personnel were terrified of poison gas being used, they began to search for antidotes. England had licked horrific wounds of poison gas in World War I. It was not without reason that scientists at Oxford University stumbled upon their own chelating agent to reduce the after-effects of possible exposure to poison gas.

Needless to say, when the threat of atomic warfare loomed large, at the end of World War II, the US began producing and stockpiling large quantities of EDTA.

The argument, if any, was simple. US scientists reckoned that EDTA was needed much more than anytime before — and, what's more, they said that their EDTA produce was far more effective than what the English had found for use as a chelating agent.

In the midst of this hullabaloo, a ground-breaking event almost went unnoticed, or unrecorded. The year: 1947. A patient undergoing chemotherapy had accumulated toxic nickel complexes in her system. Doctors were perplexed; they were keen to find out a method to eliminate the toxin from her system and save her life. It was at this juncture that Dr Charles Geschickter of the Georgetown University Medical Center thought of EDTA as one possibility. He used it pronto, and saved the patient's life — but, quite amusingly, the result did not lead to the widespread use or advance of chelation therapy.

This, despite the fact that EDTA therapy was used throughout the 1950s, to cure people of lead poisoning.

Subjects who first found benefit from EDTA therapy were drawn from a battery plant. This was not all; the US Navy had, during this time, used EDTA successfully on people who by way of vocation had acquired classical signs and symptoms of lead poisoning while repainting ships.

The results were perceptible — EDTA not only purged toxins, it also relieved those treated of conditions such as arteriosclerosis, angina, arthritis, memory loss [amnesia], lapse in concentration etc., These reports aroused interest in speciality hospitals. As a matter of fact, heart specialists at Wayne State University used EDTA successfully on a group of patients who were given up as "hopeless cases."

Werner's boon

To illustrate an allegory. The secret to chelation is in the nature of the individual atoms and their ability to form a special kind of bond. This is called as co-ordinate covalent bond. When chelation happens with all the basic requirements of treatment being met, the metal ion is grabbed and "locked up" in the chelator's claw-like embrace. The resulting molecular entity, which is called a co-ordination complex, is now extremely stable and won't easily yield to the metal ion. When this composite is excreted from the body, the metal ion goes out with it.

Co-ordination complexes, which Werner established, are formed from chelated metal ions. One example is haeme — the iron-containing non-protein portion of the haemoglobin molecule — which you've already read about. There are two more classical examples — one is chlorophyll, the magnesium-containing green pigment that plays a central role in photosynthesis; and, two, cyanocobalamin, or vitamin B12, which contains a cobalt ion.

Following the use of EDTA chelation, many more results accrued; they were all impressive. In point of fact, the use of chelation therapy was found to help patients who were declared as incurable. The bonus? EDTA therapy achieved something which was not thought possible: bringing extremely ill patients back to almost normal health. Now, as more and more successful results emerged, physicians began to collate them and make use of chelation therapy with good outcomes in a host of illnesses — big and small.

Soon enough, published articles on chelation were dime a dozen, and it was not long before the American Academy of Medical Preventics — which was later renamed American Academy of the Advancement of Medicine in the mid-1980s — was formed, in the early 1970s, to coach physicians and also promote the use of EDTA chelation therapy, especially in cardiovascular disease.

In addition to this, the foundation of the American Board of Chelation Therapy [1983] led to the establishment of specific parameters for the proficiency of physicians in EDTA chelation therapy and its administration.

EDTA has been used in the treatment of arteriosclerosis for over 50 years with good success. There are over 2,000 American physicians, MDs and DOs, practicing chelation therapy [in the UK, there are just a handful of clinics that offer chelation therapy]. Besides, the number of recorded benefits of treatment and success files proves that chelation therapy can reverse the most serious cases of arterial disease.

The downside, unfortunately, is there are not too many physicians who have methodically trained themselves in the procedure, elsewhere. This is also further compounded by the fact that the method is not approved by the American Medical Association and the FDA — though this applies for medical practice in the US, not outside. The ripple effect has been imminent — many physicians, who themselves advocate its efficacy, are wary of speaking openly about EDTA, and its efficacy.

Methods of chelation
EDTA chelation IV therapy

In the first few years after it came into vogue, EDTA was given intravenously [IV]. The method is still in use — and, popular with some advocates of the therapy. In the IV form of treatment, the substance is directly administered into the blood veins, in a clinical setting, under the supervision of a physician/therapist who has been trained in the method.

IV chelation therapy is expensive; it requires a high degree of expertise to provide benefits. Besides, it has varying efficacy statistics depending on the patient's physical status. The drawback, if any, is EDTA IV chelation is a slow process; and, also uncomfortable. Besides, it needs more than a few sittings for actual effects to ensue.

It is for this reason that many chelation therapists support the use of oral chelation — thanks to its ease of use and efficacy.

Note: You'd sure need to scout for a trained physician/therapist in your area if you wish to undergo IV chelation treatment. Ideally, it is suggested that you check with the International College of Integrated Medicine [ICIM] at www.icimed.com, or your local information resource, to locate a specialist physician who uses IV EDTA in practice.

Oral EDTA

Oral EDTA tablets and capsules are administered for their simplicity of use. Proponents feel that the technique is not only simple, but also effective. Opinion is, however, divided on the issue — some experts are of the view that only five per cent of EDTA is absorbed into the bloodstream. This, they further, emphasise limits its use. Supporters argue that this is just enough to "knock the wind out" of every toxin, heavy metal, or atherosclerotic "sails."

Today, there is considerable support for the use of oral EDTA, in the form of tablets and capsules, for the prevention of re-absorption of heavy metals during a regular chelation course.

Heavy metals, and also toxins, from industrial and polluted air, are often embedded within the cell walls. It is here that they cause much of the damage to cells — more so, because they do not move around freely in the body [*Note:* Heavy metals have varying stability constants with chelation molecules. Stability constant is the equilibrium constant for the balance that exists for a transition metal ion surrounded by a water molecule].

Oral chelation is less expensive than other techniques, easily accessible, and widely acknowledged as an effective remedy for dozens of disorders — not just cardiovascular disease. Patients suffering from memory loss, depression, fatigue, and auto-immune deficiencies have found oral chelation quite useful for removing the aggregate toxins that are to blame for the onset on such illnesses.

This is also reason enough why oral chelation therapy has become a viable, painless, convenient, and popular alternative treatment plan.

Action and reaction

In a normal chelation session, there is, as already mentioned, the possibility of some unbound heavy metals unreservedly moving around in the body. This is the "soil" that provides the ground for some heavy metals to find their way into the intestines where they will eventually be re-absorbed into the blood stream. This is also an activity, which in effect, is caused by the regular perfusion of blood and body fluids through the intestines. That oral EDTA is marginally absorbed makes it a good preventative remedy.

During a normal chelation therapy procedure, EDTA, or a prescribed chelator, picks up heavy metals. But, as soon as it "sights" a metal with a higher stability constant getting in touch with the chelator molecule, it tends to "dump" the metal with the weaker stability constant. In other words, it is inclined to favour the metal with the higher stability constant. Some experts suggest that it would make sense to take oral EDTA shortly after a normal chelation session, because any unbound heavy metal toxin found in the gut will be chelated by the oral EDTA and, thereafter, safely excreted. It is, however, apparent that it is actually the dosage that determines tangible results. This your physician would know best.

Oral EDTA capsules are sold as food supplements, but they are only available on a physician/therapist's prescription. It's also the prerogative of the physician/therapist to recommend a dose higher than what is recommended as a general treatment plan. However, it is important for one to note that the intake of oral EDTA on a daily basis is not recommended, because it can prevent the normal absorption of minerals in the diet, unless your physician/therapist feels it is necessary and prescribes supplements to compensate mineral loss, if any.

EDTA suppositories

EDTA has also been used as a suppository. Suppositories are available in strips of ten; each suppository is 1/10 the normal IV dose.

EDTA suppositories are best administered in the privacy of your home.

While it is agreed that most physicians/therapists have no reservation for this mode of delivery, some experts are of the view that EDTA is not thoroughly "absorbed." It must also be mentioned that there is a body of opinion that claims over 90 per cent of EDTA is absorbed into the bloodstream from the suppository. However, a suppository for most people isn't as convenient as taking a tablet or capsule.

****

Chapter 2

SAFE & EFFECTIVE

A safe and effective alternative to conventional surgery, chelation therapy offers new hope for victims of heart and other related diseases.

Most importantly, chelation therapy offers good hope for patients who do not want to undergo bypass surgery, or angioplasty, and stents. The big point is: atherosclerosis need not lead to coronary bypass surgery, heart attack, amputation, stroke, or senility. Here's why —

EDTA chelation therapy, administered by a trained physician/therapist in conjunction with a healthy lifestyle, diet, exercise, and nutritional supplements, is an option one could seriously consider for coronary artery disease, cerebral vascular disease, brain disorders caused due to circulatory disturbances, and other related ailments, which may lead to senility, gangrene, and accelerated physical decline.

Although clinical benefits from chelation therapy may vary with the total number of treatments received and with the severity of the condition being treated, on an average 85 per cent of chelation patients report significant improvement. Besides, more than 90 per cent of patients receiving chelation therapy report significant benefits — when the treatment is followed by a healthy lifestyle. There is also an additional advantage. As symptoms improve, and the blood flow to diseased organs increases, the need for medication is also reduced. What's more, the quality of life is improved. Result? Life becomes more active, productive and pleasurable.

It may also be emphasised, again, that atherosclerosis need not lead to coronary bypass surgery, heart attack, amputation, stroke, or senility. And, the fact remains — though you may have heard critics dismiss it — that EDTA chelation therapy, performed by a trained physician/therapist is an option you could objectively consider for the treatment of coronary artery disease, cerebral vascular disease, brain disorders, circulatory disturbances, and other ailments that can lead to senility, gangrene, and accelerated physical decline. When used in conjunction with a change in healthy lifestyle, supplanted with a balanced diet, and nutritional supplements, such as vitamin C [1,000-2,000 gm, per day] chelation therapy offers a useful and practical plan of action — and, with verifiable benefits.

Oral chelation therapy is a simple office, or home, procedure. It is a simple therapy that not only reverses and slows down the progression of atherosclerosis — hardening of the arteries — but also stalls the advance of other age-related and degenerative diseases.

What is EDTA

EDTA is a chelating agent used to remove multivalent cations [ions with a positive charge] from solutions as chelates. EDTA has been, for long, used in biochemical research to remove magnesium, iron etc., from reactions affected by such ions. Chelation leads to the formation of stable un-ionised soluble compounds for release out of the body.

In other words, a chelation process is a complex formation involving a metal ion and two or more polar groupings of a single molecule. For example, in haeme, the [iron] Fe^{2+} ion is chelated by the porphyrin ring. Porphyrins are pigments widely distributed throughout nature [e.g., haeme, bile pigments, and cytochromes, which consist of four pyrroles joined in a ring structure]. Chelation can also be used to remove an ion from participation in biological reactions, as in the chelation of [calcium] Ca2+ of blood by EDTA, which acts as an anti-coagulant, or blood-thinning agent.

Clinical benefits

Chelation therapy is the "chelating," or removal, of heavy metals toxicity. Although the clinical benefits of chelation therapy depends on the total number of treatments received and the intensity of the condition being treated, reports indicate that 85 per cent of chelation patients improved significantly, following the treatment. It is also suggested that more than 90 per cent of patients receiving multiple chelation treatments have benefited substantially — and, the improvement has been better when patients have given up smoking. Following the therapy, patients have reported good symptomatic relief. Studies have also indicated that chelation therapy improves the blood flow to the diseased organ; besides, it reduces the need for medication and tangibly improves the quality of day-to-day life.

A medical therapy

Chelation first began as a treatment plan in which EDTA is slowly administered to a patient intravenously over several hours, on prescription and under the supervision of a licenced physician. In the procedure, which is being followed in some quarters, the fluid containing EDTA is infused through a small needle placed in the vein of a patient's arm. The EDTA infusion bonds with unwanted metals in the body and carries them away in the urine. Even abnormally situated "nutritional" metals, such as iron, along with toxic elements such as lead, mercury and aluminium, are also easily removed by EDTA chelation therapy.

Yet another advantage of chelation therapy is normally-present minerals and trace elements, which are essential for health, are more tightly bound within the body and can be maintained with a properly balanced nutritional supplement.

The process *per se*

Chelation is the process by which a metal, or mineral — lead, mercury, iron, arsenic, aluminium, calcium etc., — is bonded to another substance. In the treatment, EDTA, an amino acid, as already mentioned, is used.

Chelation, as you now know, is related to a natural process, which is the basic purport of life. In addition, it is related to a mechanism by which substances like aspirin, antibiotics, vitamins, minerals and trace elements work in the body. To illustrate one example. Haemoglobin, the red pigment in blood, which carries oxygen, is a chelate of iron. Now, you get the idea — as to why chelation therapy works, and better still why it can be used with great benefit and also safety.

One-time treatment plan, or...

As far as IV chelation therapy is concerned, it usually consists of anywhere between 20-50 separate infusions, depending on each patient's individual health status. 30 treatment sessions is the average number required for optimum benefits in patients with symptoms of arterial blockage. Some patients eventually receive more than 100 chelation therapy infusions over several years. Other patients receive about 20 infusions as part of a preventive programme. Each chelation treatment takes about 3-4 hours and patients normally receive 1-5 treatments each week.

It is the total number of treatments, not the schedule or frequency, which determines results in either form — IV or oral chelation therapy. Over a period of time, these infusions halt free radical damage. As you may know, free radicals spur the development of atherosclerosis and many other degenerative diseases of ageing. Reduction of damaging free radicals allows diseased arteries to heal, restoring blood flow. With time, chelation therapy brings profound improvement to many essential metabolic and physiological functions in the body. The body's regulation of calcium and cholesterol levels is also, in the process, restored by normalising the internal chemistry of cells.

Other benefits

Chelation therapy benefits the flow of blood through every vessel in the body, from the largest to the tiniest capillaries and arterioles, most of which are far too small for surgical treatment, or deep within the brain where they cannot be safely reached through surgical means. In many patients, the smaller blood vessels are the most severely diseased, especially in the presence of diabetes. The benefits of chelation occur simultaneously from the top of the head to the bottom of the feet, not just in short segments of a few large arteries, which can be "bypassed" by surgical treatment.

The use of chelation therapy in the treatment of heart disease, lead or metal poisoning isn't its only use. Researchers suggest that there are other beneficial effects of chelation therapy, including the elimination of metallic catalysts that prompt excessive free radical propagation. Chelation therapy reduces the oxidation of lipids, DNA, enzyme systems, and lipoproteins [lipid and protein complex]. In the process, it stalls the bad influence of free radicals, and marshals the body's healing process — often reversing the damage.

Note: Though there's no evidence that chelation therapy is beneficial in the treatment of advanced cancer, there is a large body of scientific evidence indicating that free radical damage to DNA is an important factor for the onset of most cancers. Chelation therapy, as you know, blocks damaging free radicals. Free radicals are often implicated for the onset of cancer.

****

Chapter 3

FREE RADICALS

Free radicals are a large number of harmful compounds released during any inflammatory/infection process. Normally, the body can handle free radicals, but if anti-oxidants are unavailable, or, if the free radical production becomes excessive, damage can occur. Needless to say, free radical damage accumulates with age.

Major anti-oxidants such as vitamins C and E are evidenced to protect the body against the destructive effects of free radicals. The two great anti-oxidant nutrients don't transform free radicals, but they actually act as scavengers, helping to prevent cell and tissue damage that can lead to cellular damage and disease, including cancer.

Vitamin C is the most abundant water-soluble anti-oxidant in the body. It acts primarily in cellular fluid. Vitamin C is a key element in combating free radical formation caused by pollution and cigarette smoking. Besides, it also helps return vitamin E to its active form.

Vitamin E is suggested to protect against heart [cardiovascular] disease by defending against LDL ["bad"] cholesterol oxidation and its role in the formation of arterial plaque. At the same time, many studies have correlated high vitamin C intakes with low rates of heart disease and cancer — especially, cancers of the mouth, larynx and oesophagus.

Vitamin E is the most abundant fat-soluble anti-oxidant in the body. It is also one of the most efficient chain-breaking anti-oxidants available. Vitamin E is a primary defender against oxidation, and lipid per oxidation, or creation of unstable molecules containing more oxygen than is normal.

Anti-oxidants act as adjudicators in the body, and impede potentially hazardous situations caused by free radicals. They are believed to help protect the body from free radical damage. This does not, of course, mean that you can go on a binge with them. Far from it, because the long-term effects of large doses of these nutrients have not been proven. Also, anything in excess is not a good idea.

There are a host of natural chemicals and substances found in nature that have anti-oxidant properties and beneficial effects. Experts suggest that the best way to ensure adequate intake of anti-oxidant nutrients is through a balanced diet consisting of 4-5 servings of fruits and vegetables everyday. If not, a supplement with the right proportion of vitamins and minerals is obligatory.

The story of free radicals

Free radicals are highly unstable chemicals that attack, infiltrate, and injure vital cell structures. Most stable chemical compounds in the body possess a pair of electrons. Sometimes, one member of the electron pair gets exposed. The resulting compound, which is short of one electron, becomes a free radical.

When a free radical emerges, it goes on a merry-go-round around the body looking for another compound. Its intention is to filch another electron. This results in the release of a new free radical — the chain goes on. In the process, free radicals, which are, in simple terms, the oxidation products from the body, can cause great damage to the delicate functioning of our cells.

The best studied free radical chain reaction is lipid peroxidation. The term lipid refers to any fat-soluble substance — animal or vegetable. It also means the formation of a peroxide molecule — molecules with the greatest proportion of oxygen molecules. For example, a water molecule has two hydrogen atoms, and one oxygen atom. Hydrogen peroxide has two hydrogen atoms and two oxygen atoms. In other words, there is an excess oxygen atom in a hydrogen peroxide molecule.

Mitochondria, metabolism and free radicals

Almost 98 per cent of the oxygen we breathe is used by mitochondria — the powerhouses of our cells. They convert sugar, fats and inorganic phosphates, by combining with oxygen, into adenosine triphosphate [ATP], which provides us the universal form of energy we all need to live. This energy producing activity of the mitochondria involves a series of intricate, complex and vital biochemical processes. This activity depends on a number of enzymes — which, in turn, are dependent on dozens of nutrient factors and co-factors.

During metabolism, a small amount of oxygen, that is left over, loses electrons, and this creates free radicals. Free radicals cause dents in our cellular membranes, mainly because calcium penetrates our cells through them. Excess calcium — and, not food/calcium supplements we take — causes cell death and damages the tissues and organs. As this damage continues, our body becomes depleted. It will now not have the "stomach" to fight disorders like atherosclerosis, cancer, premature ageing, and other bodily ailments.

The free radical bombardment causes a typical human cell to undergo thousands of mutations, or changes, daily. Here is one classical example of the damage it can cause. If a DNA strand gets smacked and is not corrected before its other compound gets hit, it leads to the onset of a potentially lethal cancer. This free radical bombardment is not limited to oxygen alone; it can also emerge by way of environmental pollution, radiation, cigarette smoke, chemicals, pesticides etc.,

The key to having a healthy body is to repair the damage caused by free radicals before it is too late. This also means that you need to protect the body's tissue cells from the free radical invasion before they cause mutations. Anti-oxidants are substances that have free radical chain-reaction-breaking properties; they disengage potentially dangerous free radicals before they cause damage to a cell. Most of the anti-oxidants come from plant source or derivatives. They are called nutraceuticals or phytochemicals. Nearly 70,000 such plant compounds have been identified — the most effective among them being vitamin A, C, also the most potent, and E. They are articulated by the acronym — ACE.

Note. In actuality, each cell produces its own anti-oxidants. However, our ability to produce anti-oxidants decreases as we age. It is, therefore, imperative that our diet contains a regular supply of anti-oxidants, especially by way of phytochemicals — fruits and vegetables — besides a regular intake of additional, or supplemental, vitamins and minerals.

More on free radicals

The cells in our body are like small industrial units, where digestive processes take place inside the cell. The process converts raw materials, as in a factory, into energy and protein compounds. However, unlike a factory, these mechanisms are performed by complex enzyme activity in our body. The cell acts like a control system — it decides what needs to go in and go out of the cell. The cell membrane is made up of lipids — e.g., cholesterol — proteins and water.

Free radicals can cause lipid peroxidation, where the fat becomes rotten. This, in other words, is the beginning of cell degeneration. When atherosclerosis begins in an artery wall, the majority of lipid peroxidation activity takes place in the presence of metal ions such as iron, copper or calcium.

EDTA effectively fastens on to these ions, and prevents their disparaging intentions. Experts indicate that oral chelation therapy with EDTA can decrease the production of free radicals by almost a million-fold.

During the past five decades, researchers have confirmed the benefits of EDTA. They have also suggested that the protective influence of EDTA could be enhanced by the substantial presence of anti-oxidant nutrients such as vitamins A, C and E, selenium, and amino acid complexes — e.g., glutathione peroxidase.

These nutrients not only clean up free radicals, but also assist in fortifying the solidity of our cell membranes.

****

Chapter 4

HOW CHELATION THERAPY WORKS

Chelation removes calcium and copper anions — from the blood stream — which craftily augment the plaque lining the arterial walls, by making them permeable and brittle. Eventually, they are banished. The advantage — even if only a "minuscule" layer of the plaque is removed by chelation, it can improve the blood flow to the artery significantly.

This can, as you have read earlier, further help prevent arterial spasm and/or minimise and even prevent angina [chest pain] — or, angina pectoris.

For over 60 years, the concept of chelation therapy as a purposeful method to remove heavy and toxic metals has been in use. It is a well-established standard medical procedure, today, though many may ask: what is chelation; and, does it work? However this may be, the use of intravenous [within a vein] chelation therapy for cardiovascular disease and atherosclerosis, which was the focal point of the best-selling book, *Bypassing Bypass*, by Cranton Elmer, MD, *et al*, has been met with scepticism in the conventional school of medicine. This despite the therapy's impressive track record — or experts' contention that it works well, even in patients with end-stage peripheral vascular disease, needing amputation.

EDTA, as you have read earlier, is the agent of choice in chelation therapy. A course of IV chelation, for example, usually takes place over 10-12 weeks; with the frequency of treatment being 3-5 times, or more, per week. Each session lasts about 2-3 hours, during which 1.8 gm to 3 gm of EDTA-sodium is infused. In the early days, it was a tradition to infuse EDTA, 3 gm per IV session. Many at the forefront of chelation therapy began to recommend an oral dose of 1,800 mg of EDTA to achieve a similar, good effect.

The analogy — taking 1,800 mg of oral chelation for 20 days [300 mg x 6 tablets] daily at 5 per cent intestinal absorption rate will deliver to the body the same amount of EDTA as in one IV session of 1,800 mg. In other words, the amount of oral EDTA based on a dosage of 1,800 mg a day is equivalent to one IV treatment every three weeks. Besides, the IV procedure is clumsy, painful and time-consuming — not a convenient proposition for most individuals/patients.

Chelation therapy today

While chelation is legal for the treatment of lead poisoning, hypercalcaemia, and ventricular fibrillation, secondary to digitalis toxicity, it may, however, be mentioned that the FDA has not approved chelation for other conditions. The FDA *diktat* is, of course, limited to medical practice in the United States.

Nevertheless, there is also an interesting twist to the tale. Dr Ray Evers, won a representation case, in the late 1970s. Evers challenged that when a physician could legally use a drug approved by the FDA for a specific condition, there was no reason why s/he could not prescribe it for some other condition for which it was not officially recognised, or prescribed.

The ruling was a boon for physicians/therapists, who subscribed to chelation benefits and used the therapy with success. Thanks to the edict, experts also found that many diabetics and macular degeneration [deterioration of the eye affecting the posterior fundus] patients who used chelation therapy experienced additional benefits — improved and increased peripheral circulation. This was enough reason why chelation was also frequently used and found beneficial in the treatment of osteoarthritis [OA], chronic fatigue syndrome [CFS], fibromyalgia [a muscle disorder], organic poisoning, and heavy metal reduction.

On the downside though, and despite the therapy's impressive track record, the American Medical Association [AMA] has not approved the use of chelation therapy for arteriosclerosis. However, it has allowed its application in the treatment of lead and heavy metal poisoning. To add to its woes, the patent for EDTA expired by the turn of the 1970s. This led to lack of interest in research by mainstream pharmaceutical companies; the rest is anyone's guess. It is also, therefore, unlikely that any pharmaceutical company will invest funds for studies for FDA approval of chelation therapy, today, because there is not much money in it, notwithstanding convincing evidence of its effectiveness.

Writes Robert Haskell, MD, a chelation specialist: "Of all the regimens you can use to help a patient combat degenerative disease and restore health, chelation therapy is the most powerful. It produces the greatest number of benefits to the body — far beyond those of improved blood flow. If you want to get your prescribed nutrition to those parts of the body in which they must work, chelation therapy is the way to do it."

Support for chelation therapy

Proponents of chelation therapy are convinced that chelation works. Also, patients who have used chelation have been those who have had heart disease, or a family history of the problem, or exposed to heavy metal toxicity. They have found and reported a new lease of life with the therapy.

Chelation experts aver that half of all bypass procedures performed in the United States and elsewhere are needless. Research also substantiates their point-of-view. Long-drawn and in-depth scientific studies have shown that — except in specific situations — bypass surgery may not be a good option. It does not save lives, or avert heart attacks. Reports also suggest that coronary artery disease patients treated without surgery seem to enjoy the same survival rate as those who have had open-heart surgery.

What really clinches the issue, whether the AMA and FDA agree or not, is the long-corroborated fact that chelation therapy is safe. Experts deduce that there are not many medical procedures that report of no fatalities at all as does chelation. Just think of it — every year we are witness to innumerable deaths caused by prescribed drugs, hospital accidents and other gaffe. It is a long time since chelation came on the horizon and made inroads with its proven benefits — and, as for those who specialise in it there is no further need for conviction. They are convinced as to what it can do, or not do.

Besides, things have now been streamlined, unlike the past where EDTA was at times used, by some practitioners, in excess doses, which sometimes resulted in undesirable side-effects, including kidney malfunction. As time passed by and new results emerged with the use of laboratory and renal function tests, and new treatment parameters, chelation has become safer. It has also become a procedure that can be done with relative safety and ease at home, or the physician's office.

Signs & symptoms of arterial disease

The following list encompasses early warning signs of arterial blockage, or those that accompany blocked arteries. They are not something you'd be aloof or dismissive about — rather, they indicate it's time you pulled up your socks, and acted.

These are also certainly not normal signs of ageing, because as you may know, being witness to seeing people as young as 18 and 20 having had blockages in their arteries. The inference — age alone does not cause blocked arteries.

Briefly...

Warning signs of arterial blockage —
• Fingers or toes often feel cold
• Numbness or heaviness in arms or legs
• Cramps while writing
• Sharp, diagonal crease in your earlobe
• Tingling sensation in lips or fingers
• Aches or pains in the leg during a stroll
• Memory blues
• Ankles swell during the course of the day
• Breathlessness on slight exertion, or when lying down
• Whitish ring under the outer part of the eye [cornea].

Briefly...

Factors that cause atherosclerosis
• Genetic and/or family history
• Pollution, most notably air
• Smoking
• Processed foods
• Hydrogenated oils
• Diabetes
• Lack of exercise
• High caffeine intake
• Stress and anxiety

Factors that cause atherosclerosis (cont.)
- Lack of proper rest
- Poor diet, "supplanted" by excess consumption of fast- or junk-food.

Briefly...

Steps to a healthy heart
- Maintain an active lifestyle and a healthy weight
- Meet standard dietary guidelines and consume a balanced diet rich in fruits and vegetables
- Avoid active and passive smoking
- Keep your blood pressure in check
- Eat a healthy diet low in saturated fat, cholesterol and sodium
- Manage diabetes, if you have it.

NB: If you find it difficult to meet dietary guidelines, consider taking a heart health supplement or fortified food in consultation with your physician/therapist.

Briefly...

Healthy diet for a healthy heart
Dietary changes favourably influence all risk factors; so, it is advisable to —

- Reduce total fat intake to 30 per cent or less of total energy intake
- Reduce intake of saturated fat to 1/3 of total fat intake [replace with unsaturated fats from vegetable and marine sources]
- Reduce intake of cholesterol to less than 300 mg a day

Healthy diet for a healthy heart (cont.)

- Increase intake of fresh fruits, cereals and vegetables rich in vitamin C and E, folic acid and carotenoids to at least 4-5 servings a day
- Eat fish, preferably fatty fish, at least once a week; or, take flaxseed/natural supplements/capsules [if you are a vegetarian].
- Reduce total calorie intake for weight reduction
- Reduce salt and alcohol use when blood pressure is high

****

Chapter 5

MORE ON ORAL CHELATION

Oral chelation is the ingestion of compounds that bind to pathogens and clear them from the body. It simply means trying to use foods or substances taken by mouth to chelate undesirable substances out of the body. There are two basic approaches: 1. oral EDTA and supplements; and, 2. foods and nutritional supplements that achieve this effect.

Oral chelation came into use, because many people found IV chelation clumsy, painful, and time-consuming. Oral chelation therapy was thought to be a good option, or a dependable form of chelation therapy, thanks primarily to the pioneering work of Guy E Abraham, one of the world's leading authorities on chelation.

Oral therapy offers a new, less expensive, and more suitable technique in place of IV chelation.

However, before one begins oral chelation treatment, it is advisable to have an accurate portrait of the disease picture and/or degree of minerals and toxic elements present.

Says Garry F Gordon, MD, DO, a leading exponent of chelation therapy, "Oral chelation is a well-documented, firmly-established medical practice." He brings home the penicillamine parallel. He observes that, penicillamine, a drug which is used to treat heavy metal poisoning, rheumatoid arthritis, and Wilson's disease, a rare metabolic disorder, works in a manner analogous to EDTA. He explains, "Some of the benefits derived from penicillamine in the treatment of rheumatoid arthritis are undoubtedly related to the control and removal of excess free radicals... And, EDTA itself, when taken orally, provides most of its chelating activities in the body even though only about five per cent of it is actually absorbed... The chelating effects are less dramatic and slower than when received intravenously, but the oral approach has several major advantages, including convenience, potential long-term continuous health maintenance, and low cost."

Tests to be done before treatment

While most experts do not recommend the customary serum level analysis because it tends to be inaccurate, a majority, however, recommend the packed red blood cell intracellular element analysis. Some authorities also recommend hair mineral analysis — to measure the amount of minerals present in the body. One problem with this procedure is clinical interpretation tends to differ from one authority to another.

However, some chelation experts believe that hair analysis is a dependable choice. They suggest since the hair retains toxic elements trapped in the body, hair screening can provide an accurate and powerful means of evaluating the effects of collective, long-term exposure to toxins. There is reason enough for this — a growing hair follicle first begins forming far below the skin. It is, therefore, exposed to a rich supply of blood vessels.

When the hair follicle grows, toxic elements in the blood are absorbed into the growing hair protein. And, as the hair reaches the skin surface, it goes through a solidification process. This is called keratinisation. It is at this stage that toxins accumulated during hair formation get conserved into a protein composition, and reflect toxic concentrations in the hair and other body tissues. A small amount of hair is enough to establish long-term accumulation of toxins in the body.

You may well ask, what if the hair is dyed with a colouring agent, or is too short [or, if you are totally bald]? An expert knows best — and, s/he will find out how best the analysis could be performed to provide accurate results.

In addition, some researchers rely on a 24-hour, 6-hour, or spot urine pre- and post-provocation study using oral chelation agents such as EDTA-magnesium di-potassium or DMPS [dimercapto-propane sulphonate]. This procedure offers a qualitative and quantitative analysis of the amount of mineral and toxic metal load in the body prior to starting chelation treatment for the removal of toxic metal/s.

Most experts also suggest the repetition of this test three months after treatment to establish the amount of toxic metal elimination and/or initiate further oral chelation regimens.

Auxiliary measures

Patients undergoing oral chelation treatment are often supplemented with a high potency anti-oxidant and mineral formula to provide for adequate protection against chromium deficiency.

The suggested prescription is 400 mcg of chromium polynicotinate, for most patients; or, up to 800 mcg for patients with diabetes. The reason is simple: chromium is easily bound to EDTA and eliminated from the body. The recommended dose per session is 3 gm of the disodium salt. [*Note*: It must be remembered that magnesium is often added in chelation IV fluid therapy for its known biological effects. Since only a few milligrams of lead and other toxic metals are excreted in the urine in response to IV

47

EDTA, the use of 3 gm of EDTA seems just too much in IV chelation therapy].

Based on studies performed with radioactive EDTA in young adult male subjects, researchers report that oral EDTA is poorly absorbed in the intestinal tract, which is, however, beneficial as already discussed. Also, one must emphasise that detoxification of heavy metals by EDTA occurs in the gastro-intestinal tract by blocked re-absorption of these metals after secretion of the bile in the liver. This is then excreted into the intestinal tract.

The intestinal road of detoxification of toxic metals by EDTA is as important as their renal elimination. It may also be said that the binding affinity of EDTA for heavy metals is high enough to prevent their intestinal re-absorption, following chelation.

Case studies

Seven patients with increased levels of blood and urine lead levels were treated with calcium EDTA both orally and intravenously in the first study on oral EDTA conducted on human subjects in 1953. The urinary excretion of lead was found to be 10-40 times above baseline following IV EDTA in the study.

This was later found to be 5-10 times higher when oral EDTA was given. However, the blood lead levels and red blood cell abnormalities improved in patients receiving both IV and oral EDTA. Oral chelation, experts deduced, compared favourably with IV — though IV EDTA is at least 20 times more bioavailable than the oral route.

When a second study of oral calcium EDTA disodium was published, the following year, using a daily dose of 2 gm for a week, in symptomatic patients with lead intoxication, the symptoms improved remarkably following oral EDTA. The blood profile returned to normal; also, no disturbance in serum electrolytes was observed.

A third study, conducted two years later, reported that a daily oral dose of 4 gm of calcium EDTA disodium in 14 patients with industrial lead poisoning showed marked increase in urine lead excretion — from 5-35 times baseline levels. There was also a substantial increase in faecal lead excretion, which was essentially above the estimated oral intake of lead. Most patients reported considerable improvement in their subjective symptoms, a feeling of general well-being replacing fatigue, weakness and loss of appetite, within 2-3 days of therapy. Several other studies, down the line, have only confirmed the efficiency of oral EDTA.

The best form of oral EDTA is di-potassium salt of magnesium chelate. The two important intracellular minerals are dissociated in the intestinal tract and, therefore, available for absorption. Also, since the affinity of EDTA for magnesium is low, it results in the exchange of magnesium for toxic metals in the intestinal tract. Most experts recommend this option. Besides, preliminary data also suggest that with the exception of chromium, red cell levels of trace elements do not decrease following a 3-month therapy plan of oral EDTA-magnesium di-potassium at a daily dosage of 1.8 gm. However, it has been reported that some subjects show a minor fall in red cell chromium levels.

This could be corrected with chromium supplementation, easily. Side-effects, if any, are minimal — except for the urge to pass urine in certain subjects.

In another study, a number of patients were recruited from clinics specialising in atherosclerosis in the arteries of the lower extremities.

The patients were randomly allocated infusions with chelating agents, or an inactive salt-water solution. The infusions were indistinguishable by container, labelling, or colour. Each patient received a total of 20 infusions given for three hours, twice per week, for ten weeks. At the end of the study period, there was a significant improvement in the distance the patients could walk — in the chelation group. On the other hand, there was no difference between patients who had received chelation therapy and those who had received saline in terms of distance they could walk without symptoms.

Chelation therapy can also be utilised in conjunction with most other therapies for cardiovascular disease. It is companionable with blood thinners and blood vessel dilators, including anti-hypertensive medicines for blood pressure — such as calcium- and beta-blockers. The advantage: your need for medications is often reduced, or even eliminated, following chelation therapy. Some therapists also use DMSO [dimethyl sulphoxide] with chelation therapy for arthritic patients — to relieve pain and repair tissue damage.

Schools of thought

EDTA is the only chelator that has been used for over five decades to reverse the effects of arterial plaque, thus preventing further strokes and/or heart attacks. Some authorities are of the opinion that calcium should not be mixed with EDTA. They suggest that EDTA will remove calcium from the plaque located in the arteries, veins, and also from the tissues where it does not belong. If calcium is, in effect, mixed with EDTA, EDTA molecules will not remove calcium; in such a scenario, EDTA will remove only heavy metal toxicity.

There is also another school of thought. Some physicians prefer to use EDTA mixed with calcium instead of magnesium. They reckon that calcium EDTA is rapid in its effects. Hence, it is also time-saving. Proponents are of the opinion that when high levels of heavy metal toxicity are removed, it will reduce arterial damage to a great extent.

May be, the good, old Zen, or middle, path could work better and without controversy — call it the right blend of both therapies.

Oral assimilation of EDTA

Oral EDTA passes through the stomach unaffected; it is absorbed directly through the epithelium cells in the duodenum. Also, EDTA is not broken down or destroyed by the gastric processes, because the digestion of proteins takes place through enzymatic reactions in the duodenum. This explains why orally consumed EDTA does not affect the stomach [*Note:* Stomach acidity has nothing to do with the digestion of proteins].

Who can take?

Just about anyone can safely take EDTA. Since EDTA is a liquid and a synergistic combination of amino acids, or building blocks of protein, and required for proper healthy cell development, it is quite easily recognised by the body and compatible. Besides, EDTA has been shown to be safe for all ages, and age groups. It is, however, contra-indicated for use during pregnancy. It is also not recommended for use in children without medical supervision.

Note: EDTA is a blood thinner. For patients who are on anti-coagulants or blood thinners, it must be emphasised that a combination of EDTA and other medications could lower blood pressure. Experts suggest a gap of 3-4 hours as ideal between EDTA therapy and the intake of other medications.

What it does

EDTA dissolves calcium and other metals; it actually clings itself to the elements. As it dissolves calcium, for instance, it also softens the case-hardened cholesterol, among other toxic elements. In the process, you get a flowing substance dissolved in blood, which is subsequently eliminated from the body.

****

Chapter 6

ADDING VALUE

The process of oral chelation, as already discussed, can also be made up of nutritional food supplements along with chelating agents such as EDTA. This often includes vitamins, minerals, other amino acids, anti-oxidants, phytonutrients, and natural herbs.

It may also be said that certain finely-tuned benefits of oral chelation may result from the synergistic effect of combining numerous natural chelating agents, such as activated clays, certain bioflavonoids, chlorella, cilantro, co-enzyme Q10, garlic, L-cysteine, L-glutathione, lipoic acid, methionine, selenium, sodium alginate, and zinc gluconate.

Why such a combination, you may well ask. It's simple — because, each chelating agent has a preference for different substances, including mineral and metal ions.

Experts suggest that the adding up of nutrients in an oral chelation formula is evidenced to support liver function; it also improves detoxification. Besides, the anti-oxidants within the nutrients further improve the chelation process; also, they promote healing, and prevent free radical damage to the tissues. In actual practice, more than 30 different anti-oxidants are added in a given formula to work on free radicals that are formed by a variety of oxidising agents.

While it is widely known that anti-oxidants play a major role in amplifying the benefits of chelation, most experts recommend oral chelation for anyone with a family history of heart disease, poor dietary practices, or a history of exposure to mercury, or other heavy metals, or toxic chemicals. It may also be emphasised that oral chelation is useful for preventing cardiovascular disease and to purge the body of toxins that may in the long-run cause a host of health problems.

Inference: one can think of oral chelation as a convenient, non-invasive, long-term health maintenance and preventative agenda. Reason? The slow, but sure dosage delivery is one major factor that reduces the risk of side-effects. As a matter of fact, some experts believe that oral chelation could also be safe for children — but, there does not seem to be a consensus on the issue.

Oral chelation and nutritional supplements

Not all chelating substances have all the ingredients necessary to comprehensively chelate all the heavy metals — approximately 20 in number — and mineral plaque. Also, not all of them can assist the kidneys and liver to detoxify them. It is precisely for this reason that physicians/therapists have their own favourite formulas — formulae that confer a total mineral and nutritional replacement plan by way of chelation treatment.

Oral chelation therapy exerts beneficial effects on the entire cardiovascular system; it also detoxifies the body and allows the arteries to open up. Besides, the therapy makes sure that the tissues, glands, organs, and other systems in the body receive oxygen-rich blood in sufficient quantity. This is critical for successful treatment.

In terms of convenience, the most popular formulae are available in health food stores etc.,
Most therapists use plant-based enzymes. Enzymes, as you know, are the catalysts for metabolic actions; they are absolutely necessary

for the optimal assimilation and utilisation of food. Without enzymes in place, proper utilisation of nutrients cannot be achieved. Enzyme supplementation is something that will help you assimilate food and nutrients without hassle. It also compensates for any insufficiency. What's more, since they are derived from plants, there is relatively no need to worry about major drug interactions or side-effects.

Most oral formulas are available with a physician's prescription. For most tablets/capsules, the dosage starts at one tablet/capsule at breakfast. This is slowly increased to three tablets/capsules; and, one tablet/capsule at bedtime, which is, again, gradually increased to three tablets/capsules.

It is, however, important to consume 10-12 glasses of filtered water daily; in the event the water intake is less than suggested, it may be slowly increased.

In a few instances, patients have reported irritability, mild headache, or body ache. The symptoms are mainly caused from heavy metals or chemical "dregs" that have been chelated out of the tissues and are roaming around in the body awaiting elimination.

It must be remembered that these symptoms are not due to an unpleasant effect, side effect or after-effect of chelation therapy or formula. Symptoms arise mainly because the body was accustomed to "stockpiling" significant amounts of toxins.

It may also be said that some experts advise a reduced dose when symptoms of unease are experienced, followed by an increased intake of water. This has been found to be useful to minimise, or even get rid of "irritable" symptoms.

Diet and nutrition

It is mandatory for individuals/patients to abstain from alcohol, medications [over-the-counter {OTC} or prescription], smoking and tobacco use, or alcohol, before undergoing oral chelation therapy. It would also be useful if stress factors are reduced, and an exercise regimen is followed. Lack of all, or any, of these factors is not congenial for chelation therapy.

A balanced diet is also just as important.

Researchers observe that nutritional deficiencies could contribute to cardiovascular illness. While certain vitamins, minerals, and other nutrients have been identified as vital for maintaining cardiovascular health, measures of deficiency of one or a combination of the following nutrients will result in physical disease, or shortfall, in cardiovascular function:

- Vitamins: A, C, E, B-complex group, folic acid, and biotin
- Minerals: calcium, chromium, copper, magnesium, manganese, molybdenum, potassium, selenium, and zinc
- Amino acids: L-carnitine, L-lysine, L-proline
- Co-enzyme Q10

Most oral chelation products have nutritional supplements in adequate amounts to counter nutritional deficiencies. As you may know, nutritional deficiencies can also contribute to the accumulation of heavy metals in the body. When sufficient levels of certain vitamins, minerals, and other nutrients are provided for by nutritional supplements, or balanced food, the continued absorption of specific heavy metals is greatly reduced.

Briefly...

What needs to be avoided before chelation therapy

- Alcohol in any form; mixed drinks — also, smoking
- Baking soda, butter
- Coffee, excess tea etc.,
- Canned vegetables
- Chemical ingredients — preservatives, artificial sweeteners etc.,
- Chlorinated water
- Fast-, junk-food; fats and oils, animal fats, saturated fats
- Hydrogenated and partially hydrogenated oils
- Fried foods, heated polyunsaturated fats
- Lard, margarine, MSG [monosodium glutamate], processed and refined food
- Red meat
- Salt [sodium chloride]
- Soft drinks, soft tap water, spicy food, and sugar
- Salad oils, tallow, tropical oils [palm, cottonseed].

Side-effects

Side effects due to chelation therapy are rare. Side effects, if any, are minimal and/or manageable. Here is a brief review, including preventive measures:

- *Cramps.* Cramps can occur due to lack of magnesium. Best to take a magnesium supplement
- *Diarrhoea.* Too many EDTA servings may cause this problem. Best to avoid such intake
- *Fatigue.* Fatigue can sometimes be extreme — it is a result of deficiency. In this case, magnesium, zinc and potassium

— they are all minerals that have been chelated during therapy. Best to opt for a potassium supplement, if this occurs. Recommended fruits: bananas, grapes, peaches and potato skins. A fruit diet will help you get back the minerals removed with EDTA chelation therapy

- *Headaches.* Headaches are often caused due a drop in blood sugar, or low blood pressure. Make sure you eat three meals per day. Eat a ripe banana, if this occurs

- *Lightness of being.* A drop in blood pressure is the cause of this feeling. It generally happens with patients who suffer from high blood pressure. When blood pressure returns to normal levels as a result of EDTA chelation, it is best to relax for a while by keeping your feet elevated higher than your head to help allow the blood to flow to the brain

- *Nausea/tummy distress.* Avoid taking too large EDTA servings, or too close together. There is a supplement of choice to combat the problem: vitamin B6 [pyridoxine].

****

Chapter 7

CHELATION BALANCING ACT

When calcium passes through the damaged cell walls into the cells, it gets deposited in arterial walls. This interferes with the enzyme activity, and affects the production of energy. Energy is required for the transport of raw material, including finished products, and waste products from the cell as it happens in an industrial unit. Soon enough, the cells become deprived of energy. The result is they also become acidic. The outcome is imminent — premature ageing, lopsided calcium/magnesium ratios, free radical activity, local toxicity, oxygen shortfall, and nutritional discrepancy. The list is endless.

This imbalance is also the cause of degenerative heart disease, as the muscles that envelope the arteries go into a twinge.

You may have also heard of calcium-channel blockers — these are medicines that are prescribed, or used, to treat such problems. But, the medication is not a comprehensive treatment plan. They block the calcium intake by the muscles, all right; but, they do not cure the underlying problem, cell damage. In addition, the presence of additional vitamin D and cholesterol, as the upsurge of free radical bombardment, produces plaque. This attracts calcium, which only expands the degeneration.

It is here that EDTA chelation therapy plays a major role. It not only removes the toxic metal ions such as lead, calcium, mercury, cadmium, copper, iron, and aluminium from the blood stream, but it also removes the unwanted, or extra calcium from the blood stream. The result is apparent — free calcium is no longer available to produce plaque. Soon, the cells begin to repair themselves; next, the production of energy is not only increased, but also restored to its optimal level. The body's resources are strengthened, and so the invaders are kept at bay. As a result, our body is again made hale and hearty — thanks to the "rejuvenation" or restoration process initiated by chelation therapy.

Uses of oral chelation therapy

Reduces blood stickiness or clotting

Oral EDTA is evidenced to reduce blood platelet formation. In other words, it makes the blood less "gluey." It can, therefore, flow through narrow arteries, including arteries that are partially blocked. This minimises the effects of obstruction.

Improves "good" cholesterol levels

There are two types of cholesterol: HDL [high-density lipoproteins] and LDL [low-density lipoproteins]. In other words, the "good" and "bad" cholesterol. For the right balance, there has to be a high level of HDL in our blood vis-à-vis a low level of LDL. It is also a primary need for all of us to have a low total cholesterol level.

It has been found that EDTA therapy, combined with vitamin and mineral supplements, increases the good cholesterol and lowers the bad Cholesterol level. EDTA is also said to optimise the ratio of HDL:LDL. In other words, studies have found that if HDL was low, it was increased; however, no change was found when its level was already high. Interestingly, LDL was reduced, if it was elevated.

"Snuffs" out calcium from plaque

EDTA intake eliminates calcium from the blood flow. When blood is "washed" off, calcium from the plaque and the body tissues migrate back into the blood, to be again cleaned off by a new EDTA infusion. This has an additional benefit. It makes the blood "soft;" it also scours calcium deposits from the arterial walls. It is an outcome that snubs the popular notion — that calcium "influx" may emerge from the bones rather than from plaque and body tissues.

Anti-cancer therapy

As you may already know, free radicals play an important role in the origin of cancer. EDTA chelation therapy, by removing the metallic anions from the blood flow, helps cells to remain healthy. It also aids damaged cells to heal. Research has shown a decrease in the incidence of death by cancer after EDTA treatment. Although the exact mechanism of action is not known, the use of EDTA, in some forms of cancer, was found to knock the protective coat of tumour cells, allowing other mechanisms — such as protein-digesting enzymes — to destroy the tumours.

Reduces fatigue

There is also reduced fatigue in patients who have undergone chelation therapy, along with improvement in the overall pattern of nervous, cardiovascular, skin, respiratory, gastro-intestinal, genital and urinary symptoms. The benefits accrued from EDTA chelation therapy could be related to the adaptation of healthy lifestyle — chelation therapists advice patients to quit smoking, lose weight, and exercise regularly. They also prescribe for them vitamin and mineral supplements. The initiation of supplemental therapy is said to have more than adequate effect on many aspects of our life — something that experts on both sides of the spectrum readily acquiesce to.

Patients who have undergone chelation treatment have reported a feeling of buoyancy — not depression. Studies have also found them to be more attentive, with improved concentration and memory. However, not everybody agrees with the results; critics of chelation therapy dismiss such claims as nothing short of the "placebo effect."

Chelation therapists are clearly unfazed. They reckon that the feeling of well-being is a direct result of improved cellular nutrition and better circulation following chelation treatment. They also stress on another possibility — chelation therapy eliminates harmful toxins from the blood stream, the brain and central nervous system.

Metallic effect

Some metals like iron, for example, which are found naturally in our body, prevent anaemia; zinc, for example, is another element, which has a role to play in dozens of enzyme reactions. They are called trace elements, because they occur in low levels. However, in high amounts, they may be toxic to the body or produce deficiencies in other trace metals. High levels of zinc, for instance, can lead to a deficiency of copper, another important element needed by the body.

Heavy metals like mercury, nickel, lead, arsenic, cadmium, aluminium, platinum, and copper are trace metals with a density at least five times that of water. As such, they are stable elements and cannot be metabolised by the body; they are passed up to us through the food chain. Heavy metals have no function in the body; they can be highly toxic.

This is not an entirely new phenomenon: remember the decline and fall of the Roman Empire was attributed to the contamination of wine by the use of lead-lined flagons and cooking vessels? It is also a matter of concern that our exposure to heavy metals has risen dramatically ever since the end of World War II, thanks to the use of heavy metals in industrial processes and products.

Think of chronic exposure that comes from mercury-amalgam dental fillings, lead in paint, and tap water, chemical residues in processed foods, and "personal care" products, too — cosmetics, shampoo and other hair products, toothpaste, mouthwash, and soaps. The scenario is alarming. In addition to the hazards at home and outdoors, many occupations involve daily heavy metal exposure. Over 50 professions entail exposure to mercury alone. These include physicians/therapists, pharmaceutical workers, dental occupation, laboratory workers, hairdressers, painters, printers, welders, metalworkers, cosmetic workers, battery makers, engravers, photographers, visual artists, and potters.

The effects of heavy metal toxicity

Heavy metals can directly affect our behaviour by manipulating mental and neurological functions. Besides, they can contrive neurotransmitter production and utilisation, and also alter numerous metabolic body processes. This can lead to dysfunctions in the blood and heart, and also affect the body's natural detoxification pathways, such as the colon, liver, kidneys, and skin. Heavy elements can also distort the endocrine [hormonal] and nervous systems, energy production, including enzymatic, gastro-intestinal, immune, reproductive, and urinary systems and functions.

Researchers indicate that breathing heavy metals at their non-toxic levels can also affect health. This can increase allergic reactions, and lead to genetic mutation, or destroy both "good" and "bad" bacteria. The cumulative effects are enormous — toxic metals expand from the influx of oxidative free radicals they proliferate. They also increase the acidity levels of the blood.

The condition can lead to inflammation in arteries and tissues, causing more calcium to be drawn to the area as a barrier. The result is slow progression of atherosclerosis. And, when calcium is not replenished as much as it is eliminated, it leads to osteoporosis — a condition defined by brittle bones [due to loss of bone density].

While it goes without saying that even minute levels of toxic elements have downbeat health consequences, children and the elderly, whose immune systems are either underdeveloped or age-compromised, are more vulnerable to toxic element damage.

Protecting from the effects of heavy metals

Regulation isn't the answer; what needs to be done is reducing the toxicity emanated from manufacturing units, if not curtailment of production. Logic isn't also the answer here, except, of course, lead, where the use of the element can be reduced.

To think differently, if the production of all heavy metals were to stop today, there are enough heavy metals that have already been released into our environment to cause chronic poisoning and numerous neurological diseases for the next few generations to come. Some of these effects have been caused by accidents or lax policies of governments, or even corruption.

Despite environmentalists and some governments, or countries, taking up the cudgels, many practices [without a care in the world] have not ceased, as focus on profit runs roughshod over concerns about health, the environment, or our children's future.

With some governments doing little or moving slowly to protect the public from the hazards of heavy metals, it is up to individuals to take measures to protect themselves. According to conventional medicine, there is nothing a person can do to address aluminium, arsenic, cadmium, lead, mercury, or nickel exposure, aside from avoiding known sources.

Given the prevalence of these toxins in our lives, this is almost impossible.

Fortunately, there is now a way to get these harmful substances out of the body. Chelation therapy and its detoxification protocols, along with specific nutritional therapies, can help remove heavy metals and chemical toxins and reduce the toxic load our bodies endure on a daily basis.

Why EDTA is effective

Cardiovascular disease [CVD] is the leading cause of death in the US, Europe, and also elsewhere across the globe. CVD includes coronary heart disease or diseases of the arteries [atherosclerosis], heart attack, stroke, high blood pressure, arrhythmia, rheumatic heart disease and other dysfunctions.

According to mortality statistics, about four million people per year die of CVD in the US alone — in other words, this is about 1/2 of all deaths registered every year. In terms of average, it is approximately one death every 30 seconds. It is reported that over 700,000 coronary bypass surgeries and over 500,000 angioplasties are performed in the US alone, on an average, annually. It is needless to mention that these procedures are costly; they are also often accompanied by unwanted side effects, most often due to post-operative prescription drug treatment.

Note: There are a host of nutritional substances such as vitamin C and the amino acids — cysteine and aspartic acid — that have chelating properties. However, none of them has the range of activity of EDTA. When taken on a daily basis, oral EDTA binds essential nutrients in the digestive tract and blocks their absorption. This could lead to deficiencies, as already cited. Nutritional supplementation, therapists observe, more than compensates for any loss caused by chelation therapy. Also, EDTA therapy on a daily basis is best taken under the supervision of an expert.

Diagnosis of disease, including atherosclerosis

A diagnosis of any disease, or illness, is made by your physician based on a physical examination and evaluation of history. Besides this, your physician may institute simple laboratory [blood and urine] tests and call for other diagnostic procedures to make a quick, precise diagnosis. These include electrocardiography [ECG], stress testing, electrophysiological and tilt table testing, X-rays, ultrasonography, including echocardiography, magnetic resonance imaging [MRI], radionuclide imaging, positron emission tomography [PET], cardiac catheterisation, central venous catheterisation, and angiography. Computed tomography [CT] and fluoroscopy are used occasionally. Blood tests to measure levels of sugar — for diabetes — cholesterol and other substances are also often performed.

Preventing CVD with oral EDTA chelation

Atherosclerosis is a slow, prolonged process. It is, therefore, advisable for everyone to undergo a cardiovascular disease [CVD] prevention programme to nip the plaque in the bud. The first thing for everyone to do is to initiate dietetic change and improvement, including an exercise regimen, and nutritional supplements, that will not only improve your overall health but also "scour" your veins and arteries of toxins through chelation.

Oral chelation "seizes" unwanted substances that can cause LDL [bad] cholesterol plaque build-up. It can also save us from free radical damage. Chelation can knock free radicals and prepare them for elimination through the urine. A natural process, oral chelation is akin to "roto-rootering" the cardiovascular system — a process that can help the body purify the arteries and veins, as well as detoxify the liver and kidneys.

EDTA chelation as FDA-approved treatment plan

EDTA is approved by the FDA, US, for the treatment of lead poisoning and other metal toxicities when used intravenously. A number of studies have found it also effective in treating blood vessel diseases, and improving blood flow to the heart, legs and brain.

Oral EDTA was first used as a line of treatment by the US Navy in the 1940s to help combat lead toxicity in thousands of sailors. Today, it is not only used as a treatment option in atherosclerosis, but also as an anti-oxidant in foods, and as a chelating agent in pharmaceuticals and the cosmetic industry, besides playing the role of an anti-coagulant for blood taken for laboratory investigations.

As a chelating agent of choice, EDTA forms a stable, soluble complex with calcium, and is readily excreted by the kidneys. In standard practice, a dose of 50 mg per kg body weight of EDTA in 24 hours by slow intravenous infusion is recommended for adults. The maximum daily dose is 3 gm.

It would be interesting to note that EDTA has been used successfully as a topical application for calcified corneal opacities too.

****

Chapter 8

CHELATION: BETTER THAN BYPASS

Chelation therapy offers a viable alternative. A study of 2,870 cases conducted by Efrain Olszewer, MD, and James Carter, MD, Head of Nutrition at the Department of Applied Health Science, School of Public Health and Tropical Medicine at Tulane University, a few years ago, documented that EDTA chelation therapy brought about significant improvement in 93.09 per cent of patients suffering from ischaemic heart disease [coronary artery blockage].

Besides, it has been estimated by Elmer Cranton, MD, of Troutdale, Virginia, author of *Bypassing Bypass*, that chelation therapy can help avoid bypass surgery in 85 per cent of cases. Cranton is also of the opinion that chelation therapy administered according to established protocols has not led to one serious side-effect, so far.

One more thing. Chelation therapy, according to experts, is at least 300 times safer than bypass surgery.

Bypass and chelation therapy compared

Rushing into bypass surgery may not be just as good as one may contemplate. This is substantiated by the findings of a 10-year, US$24-million study conducted by the National Institutes of Health [NIH], US. The study compared post-operative survival rates of "bypassed" patients with a co-ordinated group of just affected patients who were treated without surgery.

The results of the study showed that there was no advantage for the majority of patients who had been operated upon, as compared to those treated without surgery. However, it should be borne in mind that the study did not include either chelation therapy, or the newer calcium blocker drugs, for analysis. Also, only half of the patients received beta-blocker drugs. Besides, the study was also conducted before the advent of new calcium- and new beta-blockers.

It is an acknowledged fact that patients with left main coronary artery blockage survive marginally longer following surgery. However, having surgery alone didn't improve the chances for most patients to live longer and healthier lives — as study results have statistically evaluated. The incidence of heart attacks [myocardial infarction] was also similar when weighed against a large group of patients treated surgically vis-à-vis non-surgical treatment, without the use of chelation therapy.

It is also a matter of concern that many people, who have had one bypass operation, often need a second bypass. It is also a subject of worry that blood vessels that weren't bypassed earlier develop clogs. Besides, reports evidence the fact that the transplanted vessels, used in the first graft, often get crammed with new plaque.

In addition, there is also a possibility of transplant malfunction. Statistics suggest that grafted vessels "slam" in 40 per cent of patients; besides this, 60 per cent of cases develop narrowing of the blood vessels. The chances of a patient who has undergone bypass needing another is about five per cent every year. Some specialists estimate, your chances of needing a second operation, in these instances, could be as high as 30-40 per cent, in five years. Also, the drawback percentage for balloon angioplasty — with or without stents — is still worse. Besides, you need to contend in terms of serious complications, even after patients survive following the surgical procedure.

Chelation therapists suggest that the non-invasive chelation technique has an edge over conventional surgery. Here's why —

- Restenosis of coronary arteries, following bypass, occurs within six months in as many as one in three cases. EDTA chelation permanently removes blood vessel obstruction throughout the body without dangerous and expensive surgery
- A meta-analysis of 19 studies of 22,765 patients receiving EDTA chelation therapy for vascular disease found measurable improvement in 87 per cent of patients
- In a study of 2,870 patients with various degrees of degenerative diseases, especially vascular disease, almost 90 per cent showed excellent improvement with chelation therapy. The pointers used were walking distance, ECG, and Doppler tests
- A small, blinded, cross-over study of patients with peripheral vascular disease found significant improvement in walking distance and blood flow after chelation therapy
- In 30 patients with carotid artery stenosis [narrowing], there was a more than 30 per cent improvement in blood flow following EDTA treatment
- EDTA chelation treatment was evaluated in patients with carotid and coronary disease using technetium 99 isotope technique. Significant improvement in arterial blood flow and heart pumping ability was reported
- There is often significant clinical improvement following EDTA treatment. This has, for example, been revealed by retinal photographs in patients with macular [retinal] degeneration.

- 65 patients who were wait-listed for CABG [coronary artery bypass graft] surgery, for a mean of six months, were treated with EDTA chelation therapy. Symptoms in 58 patients — i.e., 89 per cent — improved to such an extent that they were able to call off their surgical procedure. Also, 27 patients, who were also recommended limb amputation, were spared from the procedure by way of EDTA chelation therapy in the same study.

Chelation patients, studies report, are quite capable of arriving at work and resuming their regular, including sports activities without the need to undergo surgery. On a proper diet, exercise within limits of easiness, besides nutritional supplement intake, and intervallic maintenance chelation treatments, patients have been reported to be free from risks of further heart attacks, strokes, senility, or gangrenous affections. It is, however, essential for one to understand the character of the disease one may suffer from and consider all possible treatment options, before making an intelligent decision based on individual needs. On the logical side, however, you need to remember that when chelation therapy and other non-surgical therapies fail, bypass would remain and still be available as a choice of treatment.

Choosing Dr Right

If you are interested in chelation therapy, it is always best to choose a physician/therapist who follows the protocol of the American Board of Chelation Therapy, or the American College of Advancement in Medicine [ACAM], or an accepted standard, or benchmark, in the country you live.

The dosage and treatment are often set for each patient according to age, sex, weight, and kidney function — and, the therapy is often administered on individual needs as the physician/therapist would deem fit. Besides, the expert or trained staff members will be readily available to deal with unpleasant symptoms, if any, that may occur during the process — e.g., dizziness due to low blood sugar levels.

There is also something of a nature-nurture phenomenon in the chelation act. It goes without saying that several natural chelation processes in the body take place on a regular basis, and they play a significant role in digestion, assimilation of food, and transport of nutrients, including the formation of enzymes and hormones, besides detoxification of toxic elements, as already discussed.

The use of chelation therapy for atherosclerosis, as you know, emerged when physicians administering chelation for lead toxicity observed that patients who also had atherosclerosis experienced improvement following chelation. It was a small step in 1952. Fifty-eight years on, chelation has come a long way as a dependable line of non-invasive treatment for cardiovascular disease.

Over 2,500 scientific journal articles have been published on the use of EDTA as a chelation agent; besides, thousands of patients have received the therapy with perceptible benefits. Physicians and studies testify that the success rate of chelation therapy in increasing blood circulation is 80 per cent — especially, in patients who have received adequate chelation.

Cardiac health and beyond

Excessive calcium can be a risk factor for heart attack, even when cholesterol is under control. That chelation reduces calcium plaques on arterial walls is a fact you may know quite well now. However, do you know that atherosclerotic plaques are not limited to arteries of the heart? Actually, they are extensive and can affect blood flow, or delivery of oxygen to every cell, tissue, gland, organ, and system, which are served by the over 125,000 km of blood vessels in the body?

Chelation therapy, studies suggest, reaches every blood vessel in the body — from the largest artery to the tiniest capillary and arteriole — many of them far too small or too deep within the brain, or other organs, that cannot be reached by way of conventional surgery.

Chelation does more to our body and health than improvement in our circulatory, or cardiovascular, health. Studies report that chelation therapy —

- Provides constancy of arterial membranes and resiliency
- Prevents blood clot formation
- Reduces peripheral vascular disease
- Regulates cardiac arrhythmia
- Improves vision, memory
- Treats myocarditis
- Significantly reduces cancer mortality rates — as a preventative
- Protects against iron poisoning and iron storage disease; detoxifies toxins
- Improves capillary blood flow; and, also peripheral blood circulation to the extremities
- Removes calcium deposits from the elastic tissues
- Improves red blood cell [RBC] constancy; and, also potassium assimilation
- Reduces blood pressure levels, and also vascular spasm.

Besides its overall effectiveness in cardiovascular disease and heavy metal toxicity, research has also documented the benefits of chelation therapy in as diverse conditions as aneurysm, stroke, Alzheimer's disease, dementia, arthritis, auto-immune conditions, like rheumatoid arthritis, osteoporosis, cancer, cataracts, diabetes, emphysema, gallbladder stones, high blood pressure, kidney stones, Lou Gehrig's disease [a progressive neuromuscular disorder], Parkinson's disease, scleroderma [thickened skin disorder], varicose veins, venomous snake bites, and other conditions, that cause diminished oxygen delivery and blood flow.

Reduced cancer mortality

A published article of an 18-year follow-up of a group of 56 chelation therapy patients from the University of Zurich, Switzerland, compared the death rate from cancer with that of a control group of patients who did not receive chelation therapy. The authors of the article found that patients who received EDTA chelation therapy had a 90 per cent reduction of death from cancer. Epidemiologists who reviewed the data found no fault with the reported facts, or inference.

Cost-benefits

The conventional treatment of CVD is a whopping US$200 billion dollars annually in the United States alone. While bypass surgery [bypassing the blocked heart artery with grafted artery], costs on an average US$75,000, with possibility of recurrence, approximately 20,000 people die every year as a result of it, or angioplasty [ballooning of the occluded artery; average cost US$60,000]. Likewise, heart bypass surgery in a private hospital in the UK may cost about £20,000. This has prompted many physicians and medical experts to suggest that coronary bypass surgery is over-prescribed and also sometimes needless.

Classically, many patients arrive for chelation therapy in bad shape, due to diseases caused by blocked arteries. However, despite the unhealthy prognosis, results are so good after chelation therapy, that within a few weeks or months, they're amazingly better. Statistics reveals that many patients have undergone chelation therapy exclusively; so have so many that have undergone bypass surgery, the difference being of degree.

Several research studies have been published with results of before-and-after diagnostic tests using radioisotopes and ultrasound. Results statistically testify that blood flow increases following chelation therapy. Some physicians have based their observations without blood-flow studies. They contend that there is improvement in leg pain on walking, or angina becomes less annoying, and physical stamina and mental perception perk up — these benefits by themselves are enough to substantiate the rewards of EDTA chelation therapy.

IV chelation therapy costs up to £1,500-2,000, or more, for 30 treatments, which is grossly economical in comparison to bypass surgery [approximately £20,000]. This would also include associated kidney tests. Each chelation treatment takes 3-4 hours to complete.

On the other hand, a 30-day oral chelation therapy plan with EDTA to help improve your health could cost just £4.00 per month or less. In other words, it costs 1/10th the expense of IV chelation therapy.

Besides, oral chelation therapy is not only safe, it is also cost-effective. It removes calcium too in conditions such as arterial plaques, which contribute to clogged arteries, bursitis, arthritis, and kidney stones. In the process, it helps restore blood levels in the body where there has been an unnatural build-up of calcium. As

Garry F Gordon, MD, DO, puts it, "If calcium levels start to drop, the parathyroid glands kick in and start secreting parathormone which 'steals' back enough calcium from EDTA [and, other] chelates to keep the heart beating normally [serum calcium must stay at a constant level for normal heart function] and activate cells called osteoblasts, which strengthen and rebuild the bones. The more chelation we give people, the less osteoporosis they have and the less age-related calcium accumulation [arterial wall plaques] there is in the blood vessels."

By restoring good quality circulation to all the tissues of the body, chelation therapy can help us to avoid bypass surgery, reverse gangrene, alleviate intermittent claudication [cramps] of the legs, and restore memory. Due to its ability to remove toxic metal ions, chelation therapy also reduces internal inflammation caused by free radicals.

Monitoring progress

Chelation therapists suggest that it is important for one to monitor patients after treatment on the following guidelines

- Blood pressure readings
- Laboratory tests for cholesterol and other blood components
- Vascular consistency
- Blood sugar levels
- Renal function
- Tissue minerals

A whole food, low-fat diet, and appropriate exercise — including rebounding on a mini-trampoline, a natural chelating exercise — are recommended as part of your chelation treatment programme. Many therapists also prescribe a supplemental course of vitamin and nutritional supplements that also include vitamin C, vitamin E, the anti-coagulant heparin, selenium, chromium, copper, zinc, and manganese. Smoking is strictly prohibited; and, emphasis is laid on abstinence from alcohol.

The actual cost for oral chelation treatment overall depends on the expert's experience and the nutritional programme/supplement prescribed; but, by and large, it is economical and affordable for most individuals/patients.

Aspirin versus EDTA

Experts say that aspirin is nearly three-and-a-half times more toxic than crude EDTA. EDTA, as a therapeutic agent, has proven to be safe and effective in the treatment and prevention of ailments linked to atherosclerosis such as coronary artery disease [heart attacks], cerebral vascular disease [stroke], peripheral vascular disease [leading to pain in the legs and ultimately gangrene and amputation], as well as arterial blockages from atherosclerosis elsewhere in the body.

Case study

Reports Warren Levin, MD, who once administered chelation therapy to a psychoanalyst attached to a major New York medical centre: "He [psychoanalyst] was in his fifties and looked remarkably healthy, except that he was in a wheelchair. He had awakened one morning to discover his lower leg was cold, numb, mottled, and blue, with two black-looking toes. He rushed to his hospital and consulted the chief of vascular surgery, who recommended an immediate amputation above the knee. He asked this world-renowned surgeon about the possibility of using chelation in this situation, and was told: 'Don't bother me with that voodoo.'"

"The ailing man decided to get a second opinion. This physician also urged him to have an immediate amputation. When asked about chelation therapy, the second doctor's response was, 'You can try it if you want, but it's a waste of time.'"

"Through his own tenacity, the psychoanalyst showed up in my office. We started emergency chelation and after approximately nine treatments — one taken every other day — he was pain-free and picking up. After approximately 17 chelation treatments, he was walking on the leg again. He never had an amputation, and he lived the rest of his life without any further complications."

Such anecdotal stories may not mean much to medical researchers. However, medical writers Harold and Arline Brecher, who have written extensively on chelation therapy, note that physicians who use it not only advise it for their patients, but use it for themselves, unlike many of their orthodox colleagues. In their words: "We have yet to find a physician who offers chelation to his patients who does not chelate himself, his family, and friends."

A major study found a significant improvement in 99 per cent of patients suffering from peripheral vascular disease and blocked arteries of the legs. Besides, 24 per cent of patients with cerebrovascular and other degenerative cerebral diseases in the group also showed marked improvement, with an additional 30 per cent reporting good improvement.

On the whole, approximately 90 per cent of all treated patients had good, or marked improvement, as a result of chelation therapy.

A double-blind study also revealed that every patient suffering from peripheral vascular disease treated with chelation therapy had a statistically significant improvement after ten treatments.

In another study, 88 per cent of the patients receiving chelation therapy showed significant improvement in cerebrovascular blood flow.

****

Chapter 9

COMMON HEAVY METALS: SOURCES & SPECIFIC THREATS

Exposure to heavy metals can cause a host of problems in the long-term. A brief attempt is made here to enumerate them — with examples.

Aluminium

Exposure to this metal can occur from aluminium cookware, foil, antacids, anti-perspirants, aluminium-coated baking powder, buffered aspirin, canned acidic foods, food additives, lipstick, processed cheese, "softened" water, and tap water, medications and drugs, including anti-diarrhoeal agents, haemorrhoid medications, and vaginal douches. Tissues affected are bones, brain, kidneys, and stomach.

Exposure and/or toxicity can also cause colic, dementia, oesophagitis, gastroenteritis, kidney damage, liver dysfunction, loss of appetite, loss of balance, muscle pain, psychosis, breathing problems, and debility. The hazard of aluminium toxicity grows with age.

Studies also suggest that aluminium contributes to Alzheimer's disease, Parkinson's disease, senile and presenile dementia, clumsiness of movements, staggering gait, and inability to utter words correctly. Elevated levels of aluminium and other neurotoxic heavy metals have been suggested to lead to behavioural problems among schoolchildren.

Arsenic

Exposure to this metal can occur by way of pollutants in the air, antibiotics, marine plant sources, chemical processing, coal-fired power plants, defoliants, drinking water, drying agents for cotton, fish, herbicides, insecticides, meat — especially from commercially raised poultry and cattle — speciality glass, and wood preservatives, metal ore smelting, pesticides, and also seafood.

Toxicity can cause abdominal pain, burning of the mouth and throat, cancer of the lung and skin, coma, diarrhoea, nausea, neuritis, peripheral vascular problems, skin lesions, and vascular collapse. The dangers get compounded if one is living near metal smelting plants or arsenic units.

Cadmium

Exposure to this metal can occur from air pollution, art supplies, bone meal, cigarette smoke, food — coffee, fruits, grains, and vegetables grown in cadmium-laden soil, meat like kidneys, liver, poultry, or refined foods, freshwater fish, fungicides, highway dusts, incinerators, mining, nickel-cadmium batteries, oxide dusts, paints, phosphate fertilisers, power plants, seafood, sewage sludge, "softened" water, smelting plants, tobacco and tobacco smoke, electronic equipment, such as computers, and welding smoke.

Exposure can affect the appetite and pain centres, the brain, heart and blood vessels, kidneys, and lungs. Disorders caused, as a result of exposure, include anaemia, dry and scaly skin, emphysema, fatigue, hair loss, heart disease, rundown immune system response, high blood pressure, joint pain, kidney stones or damage, liver dysfunction or damage, loss of appetite, loss of sense of smell, lung cancer, pain in the back and legs, and yellow teeth.

Some researchers hold the view that adequate calcium, protein and vitamin D, and zinc in the diet, may prevent cadmium-exposure-related health problems. Scientific studies are lacking to arrive at a definitive conclusion.

Lead

Exposure to this metal can occur through air pollution, ammunition, bathtubs made of cast iron, porcelain, steel, batteries, canned foods, ceramics, chemical fertilisers, cosmetics, dolomite, dust, foods grown around industrial areas, gasoline, hair dyes and rinses, leaded glass, newsprint and coloured advertisements, paints, pesticides, coils, pottery, rubber toys, soft coal, soil, solder, tap water, tobacco smoke, and vinyl mini-blinds. Exposure affects the bones, brain, heart, kidneys, liver, nervous system, and pancreas.

Symptoms of toxicity include abdominal pain, anaemia, anorexia, anxiety, bone pain, brain damage, confusion, constipation, convulsions, dizziness, drowsiness, fatigue, headaches, high blood pressure, inability to concentrate, indigestion, irritability, loss of appetite, loss of muscle co-ordination, memory difficulties, miscarriage, muscle pain, pallor, tremors, vomiting, and lethargy.

The toxicity of lead is widely acknowledged. Infants, young children, and pregnant women have the greatest risk for harm, even with only minute or short-term exposure. In their book, *Toxic Metal Syndrome*, Drs R Casdorph and M Walker report that over four million tons of lead is mined each year and existing environmental lead levels are at least 500 times greater than pre-historic levels.

It is also reported that many elementary schools, high schools, and colleges, in the US, and elsewhere, for example, are still using lead-lined water storage tanks or lead-containing components in their drinking fountains. Reports also estimate that drinking water accounts for approximately 20 per cent of young children's lead exposure. Other common sources are lead paint residue in older buildings, especially in inner cities, and living in proximity to industrial areas, or other sources of toxic chemical exposure, such as commercial agricultural land.

Many children today have measurable traces of pesticides, a source of heavy metals and chlorine-based chemicals, in their tissues, thanks to what is now being famously referred to as the "cola-diet." Lead is a known neurotoxin. It destroys brain cells. Excessive blood lead levels in children have been linked to learning disabilities, Attention deficit hyperactive disorder [ADHD], and reduced intelligence and low achievement levels in school.

Mercury

Toxicity from this metal is caused by air pollution, batteries, cosmetics, dental amalgams, mercury-based diuretics, electrical devices and relays, explosives, food grains, fungicides, fluorescent lights, freshwater fish — especially large bass, pike, and trout — insecticides, mining, paint, pesticides, petroleum products, saltwater fish, shellfish, and tap water. Exposure and/or toxicity affect the appetite and pain centres in the brain, cell membranes, kidneys, and nervous system. Mercury is also said to block the functioning of manganese — a key mineral required for physiological reactions.

Symptoms include abnormal nervous and physical development, anaemia, anorexia, anxiety, blood changes, blindness, blue line on gums, colitis, depression, dermatitis, difficulty in chewing and swallowing, dizziness, drowsiness, emotional instability, fatigue, fever, hallucinations, headache, hearing loss, high blood pressure, inflamed gums, insomnia, kidney damage or failure, loss of appetite and sense of smell, loss of muscle co-ordination, memory loss, metallic taste in mouth, nerve damage, numbness, psychosis, salivatory problems, stomatitis [mouth ulcers], tremors, vision impairment, vomiting, weakness, and weight loss.

The primary source of exposure to mercury is "silver" dental fillings — millions of us the world over have these fillings in our teeth. Mercury fillings release microscopic particles and vapours of mercury every time a person chews — a sort of continuous exposure. Needless to say, the Environmental Protection Agency [EPA] goes a step further instructing dentists to treat mercury amalgam as a toxic material while handling before insertion and as toxic waste after removal.

It is said that there are five categories of mercury exposure and toxicity: neurological, cardiovascular, collagen diseases, immune system disorders, and allergies.

The resultant effects are depression, suicidal impulses, irritability, motor symptoms like muscle spasms, facial tics, seizures, multiple sclerosis, non-specific chest pain, accelerated heart beat, arthritis, bursitis, scleroderma, systemic lupus erythematosis [an inflammatory connective tissue disease], compromised immunity, airborne allergies, food allergies etc.,

Nickel

Nickel exposure comes from appliances, buttons, ceramics, cocoa, cold-wave hair permanent treatment, cooking utensils, cosmetics, coins, dental materials, food — chocolate, hydrogenated oils, nuts, food grown near industrial areas — hair spray, industrial waste, jewellery, medical implants, metal refineries, metal tools, nickel-cadmium batteries, orthodontic appliances, shampoo, solid-waste incinerators, stainless steel kitchen utensils, tap water, tobacco and tobacco smoke, water faucets and pipes, and zippers.

Nickel affects the skin, larynx [voice box], lungs, and nasal passages. Symptoms include indifference, blue-coloured lips, contact dermatitis, diarrhoea, fever, headaches, dizziness, gingivitis [inflammation of the gums], insomnia, nausea, rapid heart rate, skin rashes, shortness of breath, stomatitis, vomiting, cancer of the lung and larynx,. The risk expands in its intensity for those living near metal smelting plants, solid waste incinerators, or nickel processing units.

Briefly...

Toxins in the air

All of us are exposed to a wide variety of pollutants in the air we breathe. This includes —

- Carbon monoxide and lead from fuel exhaust [This has been reduced in a few countries; but, it still persists]
- Hydrocarbons from industrial waste
- Burning of fossil fuels
- Radiation leakage from nuclear power plants and radon at home
- Contaminants found in tap water, including lead, cadmium, industrial chemicals, and pesticides
- Other chemicals that have seeped through the soil to contaminate water
- Sick-building syndrome [SBS].

Toxicity and health problems

Heavy metal exposure can lead to neurological disorders, such as Parkinson's disease and multiple sclerosis [plaques in the brain and spinal cord], to attention deficit hyperactivity disorder [ADHD] and learning disabilities in children, as already highlighted. Besides, it can lead to excessive free radical build-up, which can clog the arteries. Researchers also suggest that heavy metal exposure can lead to chronic fatigue syndrome [CFS], cancer and auto-immune disorders, especially in those who are poorly nourished.

It is a slow process — so better watch out for symptoms before they lead to full-blown health affections.

Scientists observe that heavy metal overload has a direct connection to heart disease and stroke. It is reported that congestive heart failure patients have approximately 20,000 times more mercury and 15,000 times more antimony in their hearts. Blame this on mercury, which we receive from silver amalgam fillings, and even from consumption of fish.

Briefly...

Symptoms caused by mineral imbalance
• Allergies
• Decreased resistance to infection
• Poor wound healing
• Anxiety and depression
• Obesity
• Low libido, or impotence
• Joint pains, arthritis
• Loss of hair
• Elevated cholesterol
• Anaemia
• Heart problems
• Raised glucose levels.

Briefly...

> ### Symptoms of heavy metal toxicity
> - High blood pressure
> - Disturbed bone health
> - Fatigue
> - Anaemia
> - Constipation
> - Skin affections
> - Sleep disorders
> - Emotional disorders
> - Tissue ageing
> - Hyperactivity
> - Musculoskeletal pain
> - Tingling sensation in the extremities
> - Learning disabilities in children.

Briefly...

> ### Self-help guide to assessing exposure
> Minerals and toxins can strongly affect your well-being. Here's how you can effectively assess if you have nutritional imbalance and/or toxic exposure. If a "yes" corresponds to two or more of the following items, you may have mineral imbalance, or excess toxins, in your system. It is time you took stock, and thought of getting chelated —
>
> - If you use anti-perspiration sprays, lotions etc., or antacids
> - If you have had metal tooth fillings
> - If you consume seafood regularly
> - If you live or work in an industrial setting
> - If you go through the daily grind of being stuck in traffic
> - If you have chronic symptoms of any known or unknown illness

Self-help guide to assessing exposure (cont.)

- If you suffer from chronic gastro-intestinal symptoms such as bloating, diarrhoea, or gas [irritable bowel syndrome: IBS]
- If you do not take adequate amounts of vitamin C in diet and/or supplement
- If you have periodontal symptoms
- If you have rough skin, or poor wound healing
- If you suffer from allergies
- If you have high blood pressure
- If you are subject to moody blues
- If you are not able to concentrate; and, feel that you have memory or learning problems
- If you get infections at the drop of a sneeze and recover at a snail's pace
- If you have a reduced sense of taste or smell, or poor night vision

Easy chelation treatment plan

Many of us have tiny pieces of metal, like mercury in our tooth fillings, or lead, or even iron. They are like land mines, waiting to explode. These tiny pieces of metal are actually toxic, albeit they are still used in conventional medicine. It is, however, an established fact that they may cause heart disease and cancer. Just think of it. When a free radical wallops into one of these tiny pieces of toxic metal, it could cause a splurge of free radicals. A dangerous prospect. We need to do something quickly.

It is here that a method called oral chelation, as you know, comes in handy. Do you know there are a few easy-to-do chelation programmes that one could do at home to catch the free radical phantom by its neck? Here goes —

- Sustain 2-3 bowel movements per day. If you can't get it going, you may add psyllium, or isabgul [from the genus, plantago] to your diet
- You may use chlorella to remove toxic metals from the connective tissue.

Chlorella is an algae with protein and high levels of chlorophyll; it is one of the purest, most potent forms of food on Earth.

- Use garlic, MSM [methylsulphonylmethane], a natural form of organic sulphur — an essential nutrient — and, cilantro to remove the toxic effects of mercury

It is best to use garlic in food: garlic improves the body's sulphur reserves. Clove is also a good detox agent; try to eat 2-3 cloves everyday. Garlic and MSM are rich in sulphur — sulphur, as you know, is a good anti-mercury agent.

- You may also introduce cilantro [a member of the carrot family, and also referred to as Chinese parsley or coriander] to your diet. Cilantro helps "muster" mercury and throw it out of the body through excretion. Cilantro is available in most grocery/vegetable stores.

Also, you may take a multi-purpose vitamin supplement. However, make sure that it contains all the essential minerals. It must also be noted that our body works better with toxic metals than having no metals. Enzymes require a metal for them to perform their function. In deficiency states, or when we have depleted reserves of magnesium, sodium, zinc and other minerals, the body clings to these metals, and won't allow them to "give up the ghost"

Briefly...

> ## Natural garlic-EDTA chelators are available at health food stores. They are said to —
>
> • Prevent and reduce plaque build-up in arteries
> • Restore blood flow, and provide oxygen, and nutrients to tissues and cells
> • Improve heart, brain, kidney, lung and all organ functions
> • Make bones stronger
> • Reduce cholesterol
> • Improve skin texture and reduce wrinkles.
>
> *Note:* It is advisable that garlic-EDTA chelators should be supplemented with a complete high-potency multivitamin/multimineral formulation that also includes sufficient amounts of magnesium and zinc.

Legal angle

A licenced medical doctor/physician/therapist can use chelation therapy in the best interests of patients, even if EDTA does not find a mention as an FDA-approved package for atherosclerosis. But, this "holds" good for practice in the US, not elsewhere.

Courts, however, have expressed the view that a physician cannot withhold any information about the availability of other treatment options, including chelation therapy, before performing surgery. If a physician knowingly holds back information, it is truly and surely in contravention of the doctrine of informed consent. Besides, it would amount to medical malpractice, since a patient is disadvantaged of possible benefits. There is also an additional advantage — chelating physicians are free to stand firm in the face of peer pressure and provide an innovative form of treatment, by way of chelation therapy, as one of the safest, the most effective and least expensive of treatment plans for patients.

****

Chapter 10

PROOF THAT CHELATION WORKS

Chelation physicians/therapists testify that chelation therapy works
— and, works dramatically. They have seen it —

- Clear blocked arteries with remarkably alacrity, and help improve blood flow up to 85 per cent
- Relieve anginal pains — patients after years of suffering have returned to normal, productive living
- Heal diabetic ulcers and gangrenous feet
- Help patients avoid amputation, even if the dead tissue has called for surgical intervention and removal in certain cases
- Improve quality of life and provide relief from disease-symptoms

Isn't this enough reason to justify the wholesome, healthy benefits of chelation therapy? Chelation therapy also does away with one of the most agonising problems of conventional surgery.

It is a well-known fact that the relief of pain following surgery often results from knocking off the nerve fibres that carry pain impulses from the heart — which is the cause of coronary artery spasm. Also, bypass surgery cannot be just performed without breaking off these nerves. Right?

After chelation, what?

It must be remembered that chelation therapy is not an end by itself. However, the one big advantage of chelation therapy is it is compatible with other forms of therapy, including bypass surgery.

Besides, cardiovascular medications may be taken, following chelation, without any problems.

However this may be, as in any treatment plan, patients receiving the recommended number of chelation treatments, for long-term benefits, should follow a definitive regimen — healthy lifestyle, intake of nutritional supplements, exercise, and also eliminate habits such as tobacco use and alcohol intake.

Exercise

Physical exercise is mandatory for good results. A brisk 30-minute walk 4-5 times a week will help us to maintain the health benefits and improved circulation resulting from chelation therapy. Another advantage of exercise is physical activity helps increase lactate levels in the tissues — lactate is a natural chelator produced within the body.

One best exercise option for natural chelation is rebounding exercises on a mini-trampoline — a fun-way to optimal health and well-being.

Which brings us to the most important part of the book. Ever thought of chelation therapy as an option? Great — you have made the right choice. But, the caveat is — it is only you that can take the decision to undergo, or not undergo the therapy.

It must also be said, that in most cases, your physician may not be of much help, because patients often choose chelation therapy without medical advice. Besides, they may opt for chelation therapy only because it is non-invasive, unlike conventional surgery. In some cases, they may seek chelation because someone known to them has reported beneficial results — or, some patients have had benefits from chelation therapy after a failed bypass.

It is always better to speak or communicate with people — and, of course, with an open-minded physician — who have undergone chelation therapy with success and/or find out from sources where it is available. This helps. It is also the wisest thing to do — you should get all the information you want.

New study

The New York University Medical Center began the first large-scale clinical trial of chelation therapy; the government-funded nationwide study was keyed to determine whether the therapy benefits people with coronary artery disease — the leading cause of death for both men and women in the US.

Says Harmony Reynolds, MD, a cardiologist in the Leon H Charney Division of Cardiology in the Department of Medicine at NYU School of Medicine, who led the chelation trial: "Chelation is widely practiced in the alternative medicine community with little evidence to show that it is effective or ineffective, safe or harmful." He adds: "A large-scale trial using rigorous scientific methods is the only way to validate or debunk the use of chelation for coronary heart disease."

Chelation treatment, as you know, acts as a kind of mop, drawing heavy metals and minerals such as lead, iron, copper, and calcium from the blood. Although the FDA, US, has not approved chelation to treat coronary artery disease, some conventional physicians and alternative medicine practitioners recommend it as a way to lower the risk of heart attacks, strokes and other illnesses.

The NYU chelation trial involves more than 2,300 patients and will take five full years to complete [2004-2009]. All patients will receive standard medical therapy for treating coronary artery disease, according to the latest guidelines, regardless of the treatment they receive as part of the trial. Patients who will be evaluated for the study will be 50 years of age and must have had a heart attack. There is also yet another "Trial to Assess Chelation Therapy" [TACT] now underway [2003-2012]. The results are expected to provide either a significant positive outcome, or an informative null result, upon which rational clinical decision-making, and health policy, could be based.

Says Reynolds: "If chelation therapy has something to add to conventional treatment, this trial has the power to show it. Many physicians find it difficult to keep an open mind about complementary and alternative therapies when there is such a large scientific literature to support the use of standard therapy. Regrettably, this can create a barrier to effective communication with patients, some of whom believe strongly in alternative medicine. By funding this trial, the NIH is sending a message to patients: the scientific community is listening and giving these treatments a chance." For additional information on the subject, please log on to the The National Center for Complementary and Alternative Medicine [NCCAM] website: http://nccam.nih.gov/

Well, one thing is likely. The study's verdict may well "corroborate" that chelation may be no better, or good, than placebo... and, that many more such trails would be required. Call it the politics of medicine, or what you may.

Other options
Homeopathy

Homeopathy is a system of healing based on the primary principle of "likes cure likes." The word itself is derived from the Greek, *homos* [same] and *pathos* [suffering]. A homeopathic medication is a remedy, which can create a symptom complex and can, therefore, cure that same symptom complex when found in a patient. In other words, the principle reflects: a medicine, which can produce a particular complex of reactions in a healthy person, can be used in minute doses to treat a person in whom those same — or, similar — reactions are found as symptoms of an illness.

Homeopathy believes in treating each individual — from the holistic point of view, and not compartmentalise — because everyone is different. So, are individualistic reactions against disease. Hence, a medication needs to be prescribed in consonance with one's symptom-picture.

There are a few commercially available homeopathic formulations for chelation, which have been designed to detoxify the cardiovascular system, liver and kidneys. The ingredients in homeopathic oral chelation formulas are said to support the body's ability to —

- Chelate and remove most heavy metals
- Cleanse the cardiovascular system
- Cleanse and detoxify the kidneys, gallbladder and lymphatic system.

Note: Although homeopathy is relatively safe, it is best to seek the counsel of a specialist in the system for better results and extended safety.

Ayurveda

Ayurveda is the ancient system of Indian medicine. In Sanskrit, ayurveda means — Science of Life. Ayurveda encompasses our entire life, the body, mind and spirit. Ayurveda — the oldest medical system man ever devised — is a comprehensive system

97

combining natural therapies with a highly personalised approach to the treatment of disease; it is, in its essence, the philosophy of living itself.

Ayurveda is health-specific, not disease-specific. It takes into account the patient's entire personality, quite similar to homeopathy — body, mind and spirit. Besides, ayurveda also identifies three basic types of energy, or functional principles, present in every one of us — *vata, pitta,* and *kapha.* They are called *doshas.* In every given case, an ayurvedic physician evaluates and treats patients on the following parameters.

Diet

This is prescribed according to *dosha* and/or season. The taste of the food — sweet, sour, salty, pungent, bitter, or astringent — including its hot- or cold- producing abilities, or whether the food is light or heavy, solid or liquid, or oily or dry. Certain foods are also restricted; or, not eaten in concert with other foods.

Exercise

Exercise and yoga are part and parcel of ayurvedic medicine. Yoga is suggested to promote the internal fire, improve circulation, stimulate metabolism, and sharpen the mind. Exercises are often prescribed, according to an individual's constitution, or specific needs.

Meditation

A timeless form of mental cleansing, meditation, a natural chelator, boosts both self-awareness and awareness of one's environment, family, friends, and life itself.

Breathing

Breathing exercises, or *pranayama*, are just as important. Subject to the *dosha*, pranayama helps bring a sense of tranquillity and peace, and alleviates the stresses of day-to-day life.

Herbs

Ayurveda has an extensive number of herbs in its armamentarium. Herbs are prescribed on the basis of their inherent qualities, and patients' needs. Ayurveda believes that herbs rebuild and rejuvenate the body and its various systems.

Massage

Massage with herbal oils is an important part of ayurvedic practice. Medicated oils are natural chelators — they help remove toxins from the system.

Sun

The Sun, according to ayurveda, is not only a source of heat and light, but also higher consciousness. Sun improves circulation, aids absorption of vitamin D, and strengthens the bones. Each of the three *dosha* constitutions benefit from different lengths of time spent in the Sun. Ayurveda physicians recommend proper care to be taken while getting exposed to the Sun. Excessive exposure to the Sun can, as you know, cause skin cancer. Important: people with multiple moles should not sun-bathe for prolonged periods.

Note: Ayurveda is useful in chelating therapy; however, it is best to seek the counsel of a specialist in the system for better results, and also extended safety.

****

CONCLUSION

Chelation therapy specialists consider chelation to be a good option in medical practice today, even though a vast majority of physicians in mainline, or conventional, medicine do not entirely approve of it. However, research down the years, including treatment and patient testimonies, have proven and corroborated the benefits of chelation therapy for cardiovascular disease, heavy metal toxicity, cancer, and other conditions.

Despite criticism in certain quarters of conventional medicine, which debunk the treatment form, the number of physicians who are now available to diagnose and treat advanced health problems with chelation therapy, especially in its oral form, is slowly growing. This is certainly an advance — it reflects a new wave of thought occurring in healthcare practices worldwide. Add to this the transformation of medical practice due to both public dissatisfaction with conventional or "chop-or-remedy" linear-delivery system of medical practice, and you are witness to the verifiable effectiveness of alternative and complementary therapies, including chelation treatment.

To quote the legendary two-time Nobel Prize winner, Linus Pauling, PhD, again: "Chelation therapy is far safer and much less expensive than surgical treatment of atherosclerosis... Chelation therapy might eliminate the need for bypass surgery and is equally valid when used as a preventative treatment."

Which brings us again to the point that preventative health protocols — encompassing diet, exercise, and lifestyle modifications — which also embrace chelation therapy, and nutritional balance, is going to be the medicine of the future.

Isn't this good enough reason for you to speak to your physician/therapist, or healthcare expert, and consider chelation therapy as a positive plan of action for optimal health and well-being, right away?

****

EPILOGUE

Bypassing the Bypass

Chelation therapy is essentially a natural and straightforward way of cleansing your arteries of deadly plaque build-up.

Plaque build-up, as you know, can lead to a dangerous condition — hardening of the arteries, or atherosclerosis. This can ultimately lead to heart attack and/or stroke.

It is, however, a paradox, or quirk of reality, that the procedure is not known to most people.

The word, "chelation" [pronounced, *key-lay-shun*], originates from the Greek word meaning "crab," or "claw."

The natural ingredients used in chelation therapy help "hold on to" and, thereafter, purge plaque and other harmful substances from the system.

The treatment is available in two extremely advantageous forms: intravenous and oral. IV chelation has been used with great success for many years. The only downside of the plan is you have to find a qualified physician/therapist to administer it.

Besides, you'd need various sittings of treatments — 20-50, each lasting 4-5 hours. Also, the IV form costs between £1,500-2,000. This is, of course, nothing when compared to the hefty price tag that builds up for the standard angioplasty or bypass surgery. What scores a huge point, however, is while the two surgical procedures clear only a few inches of the arteries, chelation therapy cleanses the entire system — without side-effects.

The more accessible oral form of chelation therapy was developed in the 1980s. The plan is as simple as taking a dietary supplement.

Better still, the price is also extremely affordable for patients — the cost is just one-tenth of the cost of IV chelation treatment.

What it is; what it does

First introduced in the US in 1948 as a medical treatment for industrial workers who suffered from lead poisoning, chelation treatment has come a long way in medical practice. It also has had excellent testimony in US Navy hospital practice. Chelation therapy was a standard prescription for sailors who absorbed lead while painting ships and dock facilities. It has also remained the treatment of choice for lead poisoning in children with toxic build-up of lead in their bodies, as a result of ingestion of leaded paint.

It was thought that ethylene-diamine-tetra-acetic acid [EDTA] chelation therapy — the mainstay of the practice — could help the elimination of calcium deposits associated with atherosclerosis, in the 1950s. Treatment studies were performed and patients afflicted by atherosclerosis experienced progress on a host of health parameters following chelation, including reduced angina [chest pain], better memory, improved vision, hearing, and better energy. This set the stage for a number of physicians/therapists to routinely treat cardiovascular patients with chelation therapy. Steady improvements were reported for most patients.

A recently-published study from Denmark has thrown further light on what makes chelation therapy practical and dependable:

- Of 470 cardiac patients treated with EDTA chelation therapy, 85 per cent of patients showed palpable improvement

- Of 72 patients on a waiting list for coronary bypass surgery, 65 did not require the operation following chelation therapy.

EDTA: Plaque hunter

EDTA, the main component in chelation, works by "clasping" to plaque, metals, and other debris in the circulatory system and also eliminating them through the body's exclusion system.

Some metals, such as lead, mercury, and cadmium are toxic. Lead and cadmium levels correlate with high blood pressure. All metals, even essential nutritional elements, are toxic when taken in excess, or when abnormally situated.

EDTA normalises the supply of most metallic elements in the body. It also improves calcium and cholesterol metabolism by eliminating metallic catalysts, which may cause damage to cell membranes by producing the dangerous oxygen free radicals, implicated in heart disease.

While free radical pathology is now evidenced to be an important contributing cause of not only heart disease, but also cancer, diabetes, and other diseases of ageing, EDTA also helps to prevent the production of harmful free radicals incrementally.

The best part is — EDTA does not cause any unpleasant reactions. It evades the digestive system completely, and thanks to its small molecular size, it enters the bloodstream far down the digestive tract. It is flushed out in its entirety through excretion, or elimination of body wastes.

Politics of cardiac disease

While every single study published on the use of chelation therapy for atherosclerosis has described improvement in blood flow and symptoms, it is a paradox that hostile editorial comments on the therapy have stemmed principally from certain conventional physicians and others with a vested interest in catheterisation and surgery.

It must also be highlighted that chelation therapy props up health by correcting the major underlying cause of arterial blockage.

As you would know, free radicals are amplified by the presence of metallic elements and act as a chronic irritant to blood vessel walls and cell membranes. Chelation therapy removes them. This gives the push to our permeable and damaged cell walls to mend themselves.

As the plaque is removed, it allows more blood to pass through. The result is imminent — the arterial walls become more supple and pliant, and this helps for easier flow of blood.

This is not all. Scientific studies have also shown that both blood flow and circulation greatly improve after chelation therapy.

Isn't it, therefore, a surprise that chelation, which is an effective, natural, and economical treatment for heart disease, is not known to most people?

Needless to say, it does not also get mentioned just as much one would expect to in the media — print, Web and/or TV.

Ironically, most conventional doctors/physicians do not even inform us about it.

You ought to only blame the politics behind heart disease for the situation.

You need not, of course, search the horizons again to know why. Cardiac disease has become a multi-billion-dollar-a-year industry. Hospitals, drug companies, surgeons, physicians, associates, and several other people make large profits from our flagging cardiac health.

Suppose everyone knew about and used chelation therapy? There would be little need for expensive bypass and angioplasty surgeries and pricey hospital stays and medicines.

This is what vested interests in conventional cardiac care are all about — a spoke in the wheel for less expensive therapies to progress and also become useful therapeutic options.

There are other reasons too. For instance, the patent on EDTA expired forty years ago. Companies no longer produce it, and this has brought the price down significantly.

You need not be a rocket scientist to know that howsoever effective a substance is, when the patent expires it will not be significantly promoted again. Also, pharmaceutical companies, as a result, would not be keen to market them. In this case, no pharmaceutical company would fancy using its financial drive to advertise EDTA to physicians — for a cause that won't make them laugh their way to the bank.

Aggressive advertising and savvy marketing are, indeed, the engines that drive many conventional physicians to prescribe drugs/medications to patients. Besides, they are motivated by the fact that they receive a major part of their continuing education through such advertising and promotion.

This also explains why many conventional physicians are not aware of chelation therapy. This is a big disadvantage, because even if they were to recommend natural treatments, they would not because of lack of information. Besides, those who have everything to grow and profit from our present system of bypass surgery, or angioplasty, will make certain that things stay this way, thanks to their own agenda, or vested interests.

It is, therefore, high time that we ourselves took charge of our health by seizing the initiative with our own hands.

First best thing is prevention

Prevention is, after all, the best medicine — a time-honoured dictum. Besides, there are other things you could do, and with good effect. It does also not take the world for you to make small but useful adjustments to your habits and other lifestyle changes.

Exercise, a healthy diet, and the right dietary/nutritional supplements, can all take us a long way to good health.

Add chelation therapy to our list of choices, and we can all make sure that we don't fall victims to the #1 killer of our times — heart disease.

You get the point.

Taking recourse to viable options such as chelation therapy would be a small step, but a giant leap, of course, for all for us to set a positive example to our children and our future generations. This is also something that could effectively confine cardiovascular disease to the vast expanse of history books and reference volumes — for our progeny.

ENDNOTES

'WSJ' (*Wall Street Journal*) Looks at Chelation

By Amy Dockser Marcus

One of the most frustrating struggles in children's medicine has been the long-running, and often controversial, effort to treat autism. Now, some parents and physicians are touting an approach that could be the most controversial yet: using drugs that strip the body of metals.

The treatment, called chelation therapy, has been used for decades to detoxify people contaminated with metals through industrial accidents or environmental exposure. The drugs have potentially serious side-effects — including bone-marrow and liver problems — because they also strip necessary minerals such as iron and zinc from the body. But, advocates of the technique say the drugs can significantly reduce autism's devastating symptoms such as lack of emotion and repetitive behaviours.

Some go so far as to say that autistic children treated with chelation can return to normal health.

Chelation agents

The practice grew out of the belief among many autism experts that heavy metals — especially mercury-based preservatives in childhood vaccines — are to blame for autism. An Institute of Medicine [IOM] report in May 2004 found no link between autism and vaccines. But the theory got a boost last year after a toxicologist who treated his own son with a chelating medication testified before a congressional subcommittee chaired by Congressman Dan Burton of Indiana.

Rashid A Buttar told the committee that 19 of the 31 patients in his North Carolina clinic using the medication, called TD-DMPS, for more than a year had a complete loss of their autistic symptoms.

The results haven't been published, though Dr Buttar says he is working towards that. The practice of chelation as a treatment for autism has been greeted with anger by many in the mainstream medical establishment, who decry the potential side-effects and note that there are no published clinical trials demonstrating that it works.

Some contend that children who seem to improve after therapy were likely misdiagnosed as autistic to begin with, or simply have a milder form of autism. Many autistic children who have been treated with chelation were undergoing numerous other treatments as well, including in Dr Buttar's research. That makes it "difficult to tease out the effect of chelation," says Marie McCormick, Professor of Maternal and Children's Health at the Harvard School of Public Health.

Only clinical trials are likely to resolve the debate, adds Dr McCormick, chairwoman of the committee that wrote last year's IOM report on vaccines. The traditional approach to treating autism has focused on intensive behavioural therapy, special education and speech training. Autism, which affects as many as one of every 166 US children, according to the Centers for Disease Control and Prevention [CDC], is a developmental disorder that affects a child's communication, creative play and social interaction.

There is no way to know how many autistic children are undergoing chelation. The CDC reported last year that 60,000 Americans use some form of chelation therapy. But it isn't known how many are being treated for lead poisoning or other diagnoses. Representatives for the CDC and the Federal Food and Drug Administration [FDA] said they had no comment on the use of chelation therapy for autism.

Word-of-Mouth

Thus parents embarking on chelation are relying primarily on anecdotal reports through the Internet and other word-of-mouth avenues. The story of Lenny Hoover, 6-years-old, from Royal Palm Beach, Fla., is one that advocates of chelation therapy often cite. Lenny Hoover's parents say chelation helped reverse his autism. He now attends regular kindergarten. Charles Hoover, Lenny's father, says his son was diagnosed with mild-to-moderate autism at the age of 2.

The Hoovers first put Lenny on a wheat- and dairy-free diet, in the hope this would reduce his gastro-intestinal problems, which are a common issue for autistic patients. They started him on intensive behavioural therapy. When he was 28 months, they also began chelating him after tests showed Lenny had elevated tin, nickel and arsenic in his urine. They mixed a medicine called DMSA into his juice, which he had to drink every eight hours for three days, with 11 days off. He did 38 rounds of chelation following this schedule.

"We had a heck of a time getting him to drink it," said Mr Hoover. "It smells like sulphur and is horrendous." But Lenny started making such rapid gains that they eventually stopped behavioural therapy. By the time Lenny was 5, the local school determined that he had no developmental delays. He started a regular kindergarten last fall. Says Mr Hoover, "We lost our son, then we got him back." A number of Web sites and autism support groups offer information to parents on chelation. A Yahoo chat group about chelation and other biomedical treatments for autism, Chelatingkids2, has more than 1,800 subscribers, according to co-founder Ann Brasher.

The Autism Research Institute, an advocacy group in San Diego, that supports the idea that vaccines are the primary source of mercury poisoning in autistic kids, says that in its most recent parent survey, 73 per cent of the 187 parents who said they use chelation therapy reported that it was helpful. Today, the institute, which says it is funded mainly by individual contributions, is set to release a report recommending chelation as "one of the most beneficial treatments for autism and related disorders."

Question of diagnosis

Some critics argue that patients such as Lenny Hoover may have been misdiagnosed — that such children were actually at the high-functioning end of the spectrum of autistic disorders or were never even autistic. Mr Hoover says that Lenny demonstrated typical autistic behaviour. Lenny had lost his speech ability, slept only a few hours at night, and in home videos he is seen spinning around in a circle, over and over again.

Mr Hoover acknowledges that it is difficult to say conclusively which of the therapies used on Lenny was helpful. He says that the diet, behavioural therapy and chelation all helped his son, but that he believes chelation was a key. At this point, Lenny eats a regular diet and hasn't done any chelation since July 2003, when his parents decided he wasn't making further gains from the therapy.

Off-label use

There are many medications used for chelation. Some, such as DMSA — a chemical compound made by a variety of manufacturers including Epochem Co. in Shanghai — are FDA-approved for other treatments including lead poisoning. Doctors who prescribe these to treat autism are using them off-label, which is allowed for already-approved medications. Others aren't FDA-approved. But pharmacists can compound them for individual use at a physician's request. The drugs can be given in several ways, as creams, pills or via shots or intravenous infusions. Regimens vary in frequency, dosage and length of treatment.

Before starting chelation, patients undergo testing to measure their exposure to heavy metals. Doctors disagree on the best way of testing metal exposure. Options include hair, urine and blood tests. Critics say these tests can have high false-positive rates. The Autism Research Institute supports the use of a so-called provocation test, which involves giving a chelating agent followed by urine or stool collection to see whether heavy metals were excreted. Chelation therapy isn't cheap, with medications running US$100 to $200 a month. Testing also can be expensive, costing US$1,000 to $2,000 to get started, and US$1,200 to $2,400 a year in monitoring. Insurers don't cover chelation therapy for autism or other off-label uses.

New studies

The metal-cleansing treatment also is gaining ground as a treatment for a range of conditions besides autism, including Alzheimer's and heart disease. A preliminary study published in *Archives of Neurology*, in December 2003, found that removing metals accumulating in the brain of Alzheimer's disease patients using the chelating drug, clioquinol, appeared to slow the progress of the disease.

Two institutes of the National Institutes of Health [NIH] last year opened a clinical trial that so far has enrolled more than 500 patients to test whether chelation therapy benefits patients with heart disease. Later this year, investigators at Arizona State University in Tempe, Ariz., will launch a clinical trial involving 80 autistic children, ages 3 to 9.

Half of the children will receive DMSA, the treatment approved by the FDA for lead poisoning. The other half will receive a placebo. The trial aims to demonstrate whether chelation therapy can improve the symptoms of autism.

— *Courtesy, The Wall Street Journal,* April 3, 2006.

Risks and side-effects

As with all drugs, EDTA-therapy is not without side-effects. One major risk with chelation therapy is kidney failure in untrained hands. Other side-effects reported with chelation therapy are bone marrow depression, shock, low blood pressure [hypotension], convulsions, irregular heart beat, allergic reactions, and respiratory distress. Critics argue that there have been deaths linked with chelation therapy.

Protagonists argue that this is not so — and, that chelation therapy is opposed by the American Heart Association [AHA], because it would make heart specialists lose their earnings.

Chelation: Add Life to Your Years

By R J Oenbrink, DO

That's right folks, we wouldn't survive without it. Chelation is a term that refers to an organic chemistry molecule that holds a metal atom or ion. Probably, the most recognised chelate would be haemoglobin or chlorophyll, the substances that carry oxygen around in our blood and help plants to make energy, respectively.

The term chelation is used to refer to a type of medical therapy in which special compounds are used to remove heavy metals from the human body.

Certain metals are vitally important for our survival, without iron we wouldn't have oxygen transported efficiently in red blood cells; in fact, we wouldn't have life itself; the enzyme systems that burn sugar, fats and other molecules to get energy rely on metals to capture that energy.

Like so many things however, it's possible to have too much of a good thing which then makes it a not-so-good thing.

Even too much iron in the body [a condition known as haemochromatosis] can cause serious disease and shorten life. These atoms and compounds have to be kept in the right portions and balance that God created in us, or problems will arise.

"Chela" is the ancient Greek root for the term "claw." Chelating compounds literally grab a hold of metals and hang on to them, allowing them to be dealt with more appropriately by our bodies' chemical systems.

Effective detox

Chelation therapy is the process in which a compound is given to help bind and remove toxic heavy metals. Heavy metals are all over our environment. They literally started out as star-dust, formed from nuclear fusion, now deposited here on Earth. They do many good things for us, but some of them are quite toxic, though not all are immediately apparent.

It turns out that heavy metals like to hide when they get into the body; they especially like bone and fat tissue, particularly the insulating cells around the nerve cells. Once these toxic heavy metals hide out they are still active, causing problems with our metabolic processes. They can inactivate certain enzymes, damage membranes and other structures; in short, they're anything but good for us.

How does the body handle the damage that's being done? Ideally, we have an intact anti-oxidant system that's kept in good working order by plenty of B-complex vitamins and other anti-oxidants such as the carotenes found in deeply/brightly coloured fruits and vegetables,

Vitamin E helps in the lipid membrane structures of the cells, vitamin C, reduced glutathione, lipoic acid, selenium and other anti-oxidants are important sources of free electrons that help to stabilise the heavy metal ions and allow them to be safely taken out of the cell and the body.

If we're not able to get enough good nutrition or are genetically deficient in our ability to produce the various enzymes and co-factors needed, then great damage can result.

It's been documented that children can become fully autistic after exposure to Thimerosol, a preservative in vaccines.

The reason that only some children that become autistic after their vaccinations is that those are the ones who don't make enough reduced glutathione to allow safe clearance of mercury.

How does chelation help in heart disease?

This form of therapy was discovered around 1935, but between events such as a World War and low emphasis on heart disease at the time, it never caught on as much, so it wasn't highly profitable and marketable by the drug companies.

Chelation helps to reverse atherosclerosis or hardening of the arteries. It does this by augmenting our anti-oxidant system; it donates electrons to the insoluble oxidised LDL ["bad"]-cholesterol particles with the vitamin C given in the same infusion, helping dissolve the plaque.

Atherosclerosis is a problem in which normally soft pliable arteries become hard and start to clog up. Plaque is a complex of cholesterol-containing molecules such as oxidised LDL and calcium.

When chelation therapy is done for heart and vascular disease, it's given with high doses of vitamin C and certain B-vitamins to promote the reduction, or stabilisation of the oxidized LDL-cholesterol, allowing it to dissolve back into the blood stream, while an artificial amino acid, ethylene-diamine-tetra-acetic acid [EDTA], helps to grab calcium [and, other more toxic metals] and allows the kidneys to remove them from the body. The IV infusion is given with plenty of anti-oxidants to help the body avoid harm, as these toxic metals come out of their hiding places.

Extreme care must be used when this therapy is given to folks without good kidney function.

When the therapy was first used there were problems with dosing and speed of administration which caused kidney failure and problems due to extremely low blood calcium, which can be dangerous, causing seizures and other problems.

When appropriate protocols such as those recommended by the American College for the Advancement of Medicine [ACAM] are followed, problems are rare.

What about osteoporosis?

Won't chelation cause it to get worse? No, actually it can even improve that condition due to the cyclic nature of bone creating hormones being released into the circulation.

EDTA chelation also has anti-inflammatory effects to help the arterial wall to be repaired causing less risk of future plaque rupture. Studies have been done to show that about 90 per cent of patients have significant improvement after EDTA chelation. According to some experts, EDTA chelation also has a "youthifying" effect when given by IV at much higher concentrations than are available orally.

It's also useful for treating arthritis, diabetes, hypertension [high blood pressure] and other "disorders of ageing".

Why don't more people get this life-saving therapy?

Probably, the biggest problem is misunderstanding of what chelation is and does. It seems to work very well on the microscopic blood vessels in the body. The cardiologists and interventional doctors tend to not "believe" in it. Currently, the National Institute of Health [NIH] is funding the Trial to Assess Chelation Therapy [TACT], the largest study of its kind to investigate how well it works and hopefully determine who the best candidates for therapy will be.

In many European countries, routine heart bypass surgery is not done until after a trial of chelation therapy, as this therapy is much less expensive and helps open vessels, preventing the need for as many open-heart surgeries and catheter placed stents.

Chelation is the only proven therapy to remove heavy metals. There are other agents used for chelation, some work better for different metals. DMSA, or meso-2,3-dimercaptosuccinic acid, works best on removal of mercury and arsenic. DMPS or 2-3-dimercaptopropane-l-sulphonate also works well on arsenic and mercury excess, but is more toxic than DMSA. There are other agents that will bind to heavy metals; many enzymes do this. Not all of these will allow the toxic metals to be removed from the body though.

One of the theories of ageing is that it's due to an accumulation of toxins over the life of the individual.

Anti-ageing therapy

Many patients who have completed chelation have commented on how they feel younger, more energetic, fewer aches and pains etc.,

It's possible to just look at the skin and see improvement in appearance.

Many practitioners of anti-ageing medicine feel that chelation is the logical first place to start this form of therapy. A face-lift or other plastic surgical procedure improves appearance until gravity again takes hold...

Chelation removes toxins and provides rejuvenation at the sub-cellular level. The EDTA commonly used in chelation is a good anti-oxidant all by itself; this is part of how the compound works. It's also given in concert with a variety of other vitamins in the infusion. We all know that given a choice between listening to a musician playing an instrument or going to a full orchestra's performance... which will sound better?

The same can be said of using a combination of agents that augment each other for a synergistic effect. This is how chelation is done today.

A vast majority of people will have heavy metals in their system by their fourth decade. This is not healthy for us, but it can provide some good news; these patients, if tested with a chelation-provoked urine test, will show evidence of heavy metal toxicity.

This provides an avenue to approach insurance companies for reimbursement to the tenacious patient who is willing to spend some time on the phone and in correspondence with the insurer.

As noted above, chelation is the only treatment medically indicated to remove toxic heavy metals. Since we've all been exposed to these poisons, it makes sense to try to rid ourselves of them.

The other benefits are that we can open our blood vessels for better circulation — may be, there will be less need for Viagra and its cousins too.

We also have a good anti-ageing therapy that starts working at the cellular level — not just a skin-deep face-lift.

Consider not only your life span, but keep in mind the quality of your later years, this can be.

Think of chelation therapy.

> — *Courtesy*, www.tequestafamilypractice.com [2010]

References

1. Sidbury J B Jr, Bynum J C, and Fetz, L L. **Effect of Chelating Agent on Urinary Lead Excretion: Comparison of Oral and Intravenous Administration**, Proc Soc Exper Biol & Med, 82:226, 1953.

2. Cotter L H. **Treatment of Lead Poisoning by Chelation**, JAMA,155:906-908, July 3, 1954.

3. Shiels D O, Thomas D L G, and Kearley E. **Treatment of Lead Poisoning by Edathamil Calcium Disodium**, AMA Arch Indust Health, 13:489-498, May 1956.

4. Pagnotto L D, Elkins H B, and Bayka I. **Oral Administration of Edathamil Calcium Disodium [Calcium Disodium Versenate]**, AMA Arch Indust Health, 17:29-33, January 1958.

5. Bell R F, Gilliland J C, Boland J R, and Sullivan B R. **Effect of Oral Edathamil Calcium Disodium on Urinary and Fecal Lead Excretion**, AMA Arch Indust Health 13:366-371, April 1956.

6. Manville I A, and Moser R. Recent **Developments in the Care of Workers Exposed to Lead**, AMA Arch Indust Health, 12:528-538, November 1955.

7. Harte J *et al.* Toxics A To Z: **A Guide To Everyday Pollution Hazards**, University of California Press Berkeley, CA, 1991.

8. Kellas, B, PhD, and Dworkin A, ND. **Surviving the Toxic Crisis**, Professional Preference Publishing, 1996.

9. Lewis H. **Technological Risk**, W W Norton, 1990.

10. Walker M, DPM, and Gordon G, MD. **The Chelation Answer, Second Opinion Publishing,** 1994.

11. Weiner M. **The Way of the Skeptical Nutritionist,** Macmillan, 1991.

12. **Elemental Analysis,** Great Smokies Diagnostic Laboratories, Asheville, SC, US, 1999.

13. Casdorph H, MD, and Walker M, DPM. **Toxic Metal Syndrome,** Avery Publishing, 1995.

14. Crapper-McLachlan D R, and DeBoni U. **Aluminium in Human Brain Disease — An overview.** Neurotoxicology 1, 1980.

15. Crapper-McLachlan D R, and Van Berkum, MFA. **Aluminium: A Role in Degenerative Brain Disease Associated with Neurofibrillary Degeneration, Progress in Brain Research,** 1986.

16. **US Plans a System for Tracking Levels of Lead in Children's Blood.** The New York Times, August 29, 1992.

17. **Schools Warned of Lead in Water Fountains.** Associated Press, Washington DC, April 11, 1989.

18. Winter M S. **Poisons in Your Food,** Crown Publishers, 1991.

19. Zavon M R et al. **Chlorinated Hydrocarbons Insecticide Content of the Neonate.** Annals of the New York Academy of Sciences, June 23, 1969.

20. Huggins H, MS, DDS. **It's All In Your Head: The Link Between Mercury Amalgams and Illness,** Avery Publishing, 1993.

21. Dental Group Agrees with FDA and EPA on Issue of Toxic Mercury. Townsend Letter for Doctors, November 1990.

22. Walker M, DPM, and Shah H, MD. **Everything You Should Know About Chelation Therapy,** Keats Publishing, 1995.

23. Werbach, MD. **Nutritional Influence on Illness,** Third Line Press, 1993.

24. **Toxic Elements,** Great Smokies Diagnostic Laboratories, Asheville, SC, US, 1998.

25. Golan R, MD. **Optimal Wellness,** Ballantine Books, 1995.

26. Brown P, and Mikkelsen E. **No Safe Place: Toxic Waste, Leukemia, and Community Action,** University of California Press, 1990.

27. Needleman H, MD, Landrigan P, MD. **Raising Children Toxic Free — How to Keep Your Child Safe From Lead, Asbestos, Pesticides, and Other Environmental Hazards,** Farrar, Straus & Giroux Publishing, 1994.

28. Foreman H. **Toxic Side-Effects of EDTA,** J Chron Dis 16, 319-323, 1963.

29. Olszewer E, and Carter J. **EDTA Chelation Therapy: A Retrospective Study of 2,870 Patients,** Journal of Advancement in Medicine; Special Issue, 2:1-2, 197-211, 1989.

30. Goldberg B, and the Editors of Alternative Medicine Digest. **Alternative Medicine Guide to Heart Disease,** Future Medicine Publishing, 1997.

31. McDonagh E *et al.* **An Oculocerebrovasculometric Analysis of the Improvement in Arterial Stenosis**

following EDTA Chelation Therapy. Journal of Advancement in Medicine; Special Issue, 2:1-2, 155-166, 1989.

32. Casdorph H, MD. EDTA Chelation Therapy: Efficacy in Brain Disorders. Journal of Advancement in Medicine; Special Issue 2:1-2, 131-153, 1989.

33. Alsleben H, MD, and Shute W, MD. How to Survive the New Health Catastrophes, Survival Publications, 1973.

34. Freeman R. Reversible Myocarditis Due to Chronic Lead Poisoning in Childhood. Arch Dis Child 40, 389-93, 1965.

35. Zelis R et al. Effects of Hyperlipoproteinanemias and their Treatment on the Peripheral Circulation, J Clin Invest, 49, 1007, 1970.

36. Schroeder H, and Perry H, Jr. Anti-hypertensive Effects of Binding Agents. J Lab Clin Med, 46, 416, 1955.

37. Shin Y. Cross-linking of Elastin in Human Atherosclerotic Aortas. Lab Invest, 25, 121, 1971.

38. Jacob H. Pathologic States of Erythrocyte Membrane, University of Minnesota, Hospital Practice, 47-9, December 1974.

39. Soffer A et al. Myocardial Response to Chelation. Br Heart J, 23, 690-94, 1961.

40. Walker M, DPM. The Chelation Way, Avery Publishing Group, 1990.

41. Rath M, MD. Eradicating Heart Disease [Matthias Rath, MD; Copyright 1993].

42. CASS Principle Investigators and Associates. Myocardial Infarction and Mortality in the Coronary Artery Surgery

Study [CASS] Randomised Trial, New England Journal of Medicine, 310:12, 750-758, March 1984.

43. Goldberg B, and the Editors of Alternative Medicine Digest. **Alternative Medicine Guide to Heart Disease**, Future Medicine Publishing, 1997.

44. Strauts Z, MD. Correspondence Re: **Berkeley Wellness Letter and Chelation Therapy.** Townsend Letter for Doctors, 106, 382-83, May 1992.

45. Gordon G, MD, DO. **Chelation Therapy, Life Enhancement**, 32, 9-10, April 1997.

46. Lamar, P. Calcium **Chelation of Atherosclerosis — Nine Years**, Clinical Experience. Fourteenth Annual Meeting, American College of Angiology, 1968.

47. Brecher, Harold and Arline. **Forty Something Forever: A Consumer's Guide to Chelation Therapy and Other Heart-Savers**, Healthsavers Press, 1992.

48. Halstead B, MD. **The Scientific Basis of EDTA Chelation Therapy, Summarized in Life Enhancement**, February 1998.

49. Garlic-EDTA **Chelator.**
www. life-enhancement.com/garlicEDTA.htm

50. **Urinalysis Studies**, Maile Pouls PhD, and Greg Pouls, D C, 1998.

51. Cranton E, MD. *Bypassing Bypass*, Medex Publishers, 1993.

52. Balch James, MD, and Balch Phyllis. **Prescription for Nutritional Healing**, Avery Publishing, 1997.

53. Blaylock R, MD. **Excititoxins, The Taste That Kills**, Health Press, 1997.

54. Klinghardt D, MD, PhD. **Migraines, Seizures, and Mercury Toxicity.** Alternative Medicine Digest, December-January 1997-98.

55. Klinghardt, D, MD, PhD. **Amalgam/Mercury Detox as a Treatment for Chronic Viral, Bacterial, and Fungal Illnesses,** Annual Meeting of the International and American Academy of Clinical Nutrition, San Diego, CA, US, September 1996.

56. Schauss A, PhD. **Minerals and Human Health: The Rationale for Optimal and Balanced Trace Element Levels,** Life Sciences Press, 1995.

57. Trowbridge J P, MD, and Walker M. **The Healing Powers of Chelation Therapy,** New Way of Life, 1992.

58. Nidamboor R, **Chelation Therapy,** HealthyNewAge, 2007.

Resources

American Board of Chelation Therapy
Website: www.abcmt.org

Worldwide Health Centre
Website: http://www.worldwidehealthcenter.net

Breakspear Medical Group Ltd, UK
Website: http://www.breakspearmedical.com

First Vitality International Ltd, UK
Website: http://www.1stvitality.co.uk

The Henry Spink Foundation, UK
Website: http://www.henryspink.org/chelation_therapy.htm

American College of Advancement in Medicine
E-mail: info@acam.org

HealthWorld Online, Inc.,
Website: http://www.healthy.net/clinic/therapy/chelat/

Environmental Health & Complementary Medicine
Website: http://www.HealthAllWays.com

IPC Heart Care [India]
Website: http://www.ipc-india.com

Optimal Health Medical, LLC
Website: http://www.drsobo.com

RESOURCES

Dr Bruce Shelton
Website: www.drbruceshelton.com

Dr R J Oenbrink
Website: www.tequestafamilypractice.com

Glossary

- *ADHD* [attention deficit hyperactivity disorder]. A mental disorder, in childhood, characterised by developmentally inappropriate distraction, impulsiveness, and varying degrees of hyperactivity.

- *Allergy.* A misguided reaction to foreign substance/s by the immune system.

- *Alzheimer's disease.* A progressive neurological disease of the brain that leads to irreversible loss of neurons and dementia [mental deterioration].

- *Angioplasty.* Reconstruction of a blood vessel in the heart.

- *Anxiety.* A feeling of apprehension and fear accompanied by physical symptoms such as palpitation, sweating, and stress.

- *Atherosclerosis.* Hardening and thickening of the walls of the arteries that can lead to heart attack.

- *Arthritis.* Inflammation of the joint.

- *Bile.* Bile is a yellow-green fluid that is made by the liver, and stored in the gallbladder; it helps digest fat.

- *Blood clot.* Blood that has been converted from a liquid to a solid state. It is also called thrombus.

- *Bursitis.* Inflammation of the bursa, a closed sac or envelope lined with synovial membrane and containing fluid.

- *Bypass.* A surgical procedure that helps shunt blood from the aorta to branches of the coronary arteries, in order to increase the flow beyond the local obstruction.

- *Cancer.* An abnormal growth of cells which tends to proliferate in an uncontrolled manner; in some cases, they spread [metastasise].

- *Chelation.* A complex formation involving a metal ion and two or more polar groupings of a single molecule; it is a simple form of non-invasive treatment that not only reverses and slows down the progression of atherosclerosis, but also stalls the development of age-related and other degenerative diseases.

- *Cholesterol.* The most abundant steroid present in bile and gallstones, and food, especially rich in animal fats. Cholesterol circulates in the plasma complexed to proteins of various densities. It plays a critical role in the causation of atherosclerotic plaques in arteries.

- *Diabetes.* A metabolic disease in which carbohydrate utilisation is reduced and that of lipid and protein enhanced.

- *Depression.* A sinking of spirits so as to constitute a clinically discernible condition.

- *EDTA.* Ethylene-diamine-tetra-acetic acid, a chelating agent used to remove multivalent cations from solution as chelates and also arterial plaques.

- *Epidemiology.* The study of populations in order to determine the frequency and distribution of disease and measure risks.

- *Free radicals.* A large number of harmful compounds released during any inflammatory/infection process.

- *Hormone.* A chemical substance produced in the body that controls and regulates the activity of certain cells or organs.

- *Hypertension.* High blood pressure, or repeatedly elevated blood pressure.

- *Immunity.* The condition of being immune. This can be natural, or conferred by a previous infection, or immunisation.

- *Joint.* A joint is the area where two bones are attached for the purpose of motion of body parts. A joint is usually formed of fibrous connective tissue and cartilage.

- *Obesity.* The state of being well above one's normal weight.

- *Osteoporosis.* Thinning of the bones with reduction in bone mass due to depletion of calcium and bone protein. The condition predisposes a person to fractures.

- *Parkinson's disease.* A neurological syndrome usually resulting from deficiency of the neurotransmitter dopamine as the consequence of degenerative, vascular, or inflammatory changes in the basal ganglia. The disease is characterised by rhythmical muscular tremors, rigidity of movement etc.,

- *Virus.* A virus is a micro-organism smaller than bacteria. Viruses cannot grow or reproduce apart from a living cell. [Bacteria multiply by cell division].

- *Vitamins.* One of a group of organic substances, present in minute amounts in natural food, essential for normal metabolism. Inadequate amounts of vitamins in the diet may cause deficiency diseases.

- *X-ray.* a]. High-energy radiation with waves shorter than those of visible light. X-rays possess the properties of penetrating most substances and acting on a photographic film, or plate [radiography]. b]. In low doses, X-rays are used for making images that help to diagnose disease.

Index

NATURE'S HEALTH SECRETS

NATURE'S HEALTH SECRETS SEA MEDICINE CHEST

Rajgopal Nidamboor

IMPROVING HEALTH THROUGH NATURAL SEA REMEDIES

Researchers suggest that the sea and ocean could become our new, big frontiers for deriving medicines in the 21st century. You name it — shark cartilage, shark liver oil, cod, or fish oils, mussel, sea cucumber, seaweed, oyster, shrimp, sponge etc., They are curative medicines. They are natural. They are available in profusion. Most importantly, they provide through their use a great degree of safety — for our optimal health and well-being, without the dangerous side-effects of conventional medications.

The best part — sea cure is risk-free and sure, so much so you will wonder why you have not tried some of its wholesome miracles yet! Not just a book, but a one-stop guide to expand on your health information-base — with the latest knowledge available on sea medicines — to lead healthy and vibrant lives.

Order Direct www.emeraldpublishing.co.uk
Or from all bookshops

ISBN 9781847161673
£9.99

OTHER TITLES IN THE NATURE'S HEALTH SECRETS
SERIES

NATURE'S HEALTH SECRETS

REVERSING
OSTEOARTHRITIS

Rajgopal Nidamboor

A GROUNDBREAKING BOOK TO PREVENT, TREAT, AND 'TURN-AROUND' OSTEOARTHRITIS, NATURALLY...

Osteoarthritis is a major joint disorder. It affects millions of people world-wide — and, could affect many more — including YOU! There is no easy answer — much less a cure for osteoarthritis, because conventional or prescription medications have nothing much to offer, much less to repair, or rebuild, an osteoarthritic joint. Besides, they tend to have a host of side effects — some of them serious. Glucosamine and chondroitin are natural dietary supplements, or "nutrients." They have health-promoting, disease-preventing, and therapeutic properties. They also get to the "source" of the osteoarthritic problem, and revamp joint cartilage — safely. Isn't this enough reason for you to try them out [along with other natural herbs and options] — to bring back the smile to your joint/s and promote good health and well-being, naturally and gently?

Order Direct www.emeraldpublishing.co.uk
Or from all bookshops

ISBN 9781847161666
£9.99

NATURE'S HEALTH SECRETS

NATURE'S ASPIRIN

Rajgopal Nidamboor

A PRACTICAL, UP-TO-THE-MINUTE BOOK ON ASPIRIN-LIKE NATURAL HERBS TO COMBAT PAIN & ILLNESS

Call it the "herbal aspirin" effect, or what you may, natural herbs provide us a holistic medicinal tool-kit for optimal health and well-being. They offer us the means to combat pain and other illnesses, without the adverse side- or after-effects of traditional, or conventional, non-steroidal anti-inflammatory drugs [NSAIDs]. This is not all. With the "demise" of the once-popular coxib drugs, such as Vioxx, due to their deleterious effects on the heart, the "climate," or need, for natural herbal remedies, to fill the gap, has never been more pronounced. *Nature's Aspirin* explores what herbs, in the form of simple but profound kitchen remedies, such as green tea, ginger, turmeric, holy basil, rosemary etc., hold for us — a mirror to the future of pain relief, including prevention and treatment of a host of other disorders… such as cancer. Natural herbs, it is rightly said, nurture our need for a safe and gentle treatment plan, or option — without the side-effects of conventional medications.

Order Direct www.emeraldpublishing.co.uk
Or from all bookshops

ISBN 9781847161680

£9.99

Emerald Publishing
www.emeraldpublishing.co.uk

106 Ladysmith Road
Brighton BN2 4EG

Other titles in the Emerald Series:

For details of the above titles published by Emerald, and how to order, go to:

www.emeraldpublishing.co.uk